Step by Step . . . Day by Day . . . You Will Become More and More Hopeful That You Really Can Quit. For Good.

This groundbreaking program will guide you to success. All smokers have tried to quit at one time or another—they just haven't been counseled on *how* to quit, and then *how* to cope without cigarettes. *YOU CAN STOP SMOKING* goes well beyond the act of quitting; it eliminates the pain of addiction withdrawal and deals with other physical, social, emotional and psychological issues, both before and after you quit. It's easy to quit. The trick is to *stay quit*.

YOU CAN STOP SMOKING also discusses:

- **Smokers' 5 Fears of Quitting.** Why, psychologically, you may feel defensive about your smoking.
- **Costs.** With the threat of increased cigarette taxes, you will eliminate a major expense from your life. Reward yourself with the savings!
- **Children.** Learn how to keep your children clear of cigarettes, even if the adults in your household continue to smoke.
- **Cigars, pipes and chewing tobacco.** Discover how to break these similar, but unique, habits.
- **Groups.** A special curriculum is available for therapists, doctors, human resources departments and leaders of self-help groups.

"Read each chapter as if your life depends on it—because it does. It worked for me!"

—T. George Harris, founder and former editor-in-chief, *American Health* and *Psychology Today*

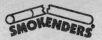

SMOKENDERS®

YOU CAN STOP SMOKING

NEWLY EXPANDED AND UPDATED

JACQUELYN ROGERS

POCKET BOOKS

New York   London   Toronto   Sydney   Tokyo   Singapore

An *Original* Publication of POCKET BOOKS

POCKET BOOKS, a division of Simon & Schuster Inc.
1230 Avenue of the Americas, New York, NY 10020

ISBN: 0-671-52303-1

First Pocket Books printing March 1995

10 9 8 7 6 5 4 3 2 1

POCKET and colophon are registered trademarks of Simon & Schuster Inc.

Printed in the U.S.A.

To my husband, Jon, for his love and unwavering support;

To our children, Joan, Jim, Lilla and Peter, for cheering me on and encouraging me to make my contribution.

Without them, I'd still be smoking.

Acknowledgments

How can I possibly express my thanks to the thousands of wonderful people who have helped me gain knowledge, develop experience and guide my days so that I might be in a position to write this book? First I should thank all the smokers who have become SmokEnders and have told me their stories; then all the fine people who have worked with me since 1969 to help deliver the program and who have supported my fantasy of creating a non-smoking epidemic; and finally, all those who actually propelled this book from concept to deadline.

I will hope that all who have shared our work and have made a contribution to my knowledge and effort will know that I am grateful and that I offer my sincere thanks.

And to those who helped with this book I want to express special thanks. To Harriet Pilpel for her gracious guidance; to Barbara Davidson and Lois Rafalko for their talented assistance; to Ruth Strine and Eileen Gill for their diplomacy, scheduling wizardry and devotion; and to my editors, Alice Mayhew, Pam Dorman and Julie Rubenstein, whose expertise and professionalism were necessary and appreciated.

J.R.

manager announced that smoking will be prohibited next month. He can either quit smoking or go outside to smoke. With his heavy workload due to personal committee

Publisher's Note

With the development of SmokEnders as both a movement and a business enterprise in 1969, Jacquelyn Rogers established what is today an international phenomenon. She and her husband, Jon, a practicing dentist, believed they could revolutionize the attitude toward smoking in this country by offering a truly effective means of quitting smoking which they had developed to "cure" Jackie of her twenty-two-year addiction. They started on an ambitious campaign to develop both the health-care delivery system for their method and a consistently reliable means of providing it to the general public on a mass basis.

Now hailed by physicians and health agencies, the Smok-Ender method has stood the test of time. As of this writing, over one million smokers have benefited from the program, from coast to coast and in Canada, Europe, Africa, Australia and Japan; this supports the Rogerses' conviction that smokers would be anxious to quit if they knew how.

A wife and mother of four children and four grandchildren, Jacquelyn Rogers began her study of the smoking problem shortly after she married in 1949. Her husband objected to her smoking, and she began to inquire informally into all the available quitting methods and techniques. Finally, in 1968, she prepared a formal research project that was designed to develop an effective method to free herself from her compulsive habit. This book is based on the central principle of SmokEnders: you face in the right direction to quit smoking by careful preparation, by developing the right attitude and by knowing you're worth the benefits. It reflects Mrs. Rogers' knowledge and experience, gained through twenty-five years of working with smokers and a twenty-two-year history, which preceded it, of being a smoker and trying to quit. Mrs. Rogers moved from trial and error to analysis of the data and thus to the most successful method for stopping smoking yet devised.

Contents

Preface

Things have certainly changed since I sat down to write this book in 1977—and even since I updated it in 1987.

Smoking was socially acceptable. (Non-smokers were viewed as weird. Out of the mainstream. Quitters were viewed as "chicken"—sort of an admission that the fear of cancer made them quit.) Now smokers are in the minority. Smoking is considered déclassé. Smokers tell me their biggest reason for quitting is "because I'm embarrassed to smoke." Another view is, "It's too much of a hassle to smoke anymore . . ." Of the fifty million smokers in the USA, most want to quit, according to U.S. government studies. Unfortunately, they don't know how to quit. That's what this book is about:

IT'S A PROVEN COURSE IN MOTIVATING PEOPLE TO QUIT SMOKING AND THEN GENTLY LEADING THEM TO SUCCESS. AND IT REALLY DOES WHAT IT SAYS IT WILL DO—ONE EASY, COMFORTABLE STEP AT A TIME!

THE JOY IS—YOU SMOKE WHILE YOU LEARN TO QUIT. YOU'LL BE GENTLY DETOXIFIED *BEFORE* YOU QUIT, SO YOU WON'T CLIMB THE WALLS. AND YOU'LL DISCONNECT ALL THE EMOTIONAL AND PSYCHOLOGICAL CONNECTIONS *BEFORE* YOU QUIT, SO YOU CAN STOP SMOKING PERMANENTLY.

After all, it's easy to quit. It's hard to *stay* quit.

Back in 1968, when I finally attacked my smoking habit and created this method for me, smoking wasn't considered addictive. It was classified as "habituative." We smokers all knew we were hooked, that something in our cigarettes was addictive, but the tobacco lobby was very strong—until

1994. During congressional hearings we were not surprised to learn that the cigarette makers lied to us: they knew nicotine was addictive in the fifties, but they hid their research. (*N.Y. Times* 6/18/94)

Pity the poor, billion-dollar-a-year cigarette industry. How could they market their product as something that made you appear more sexy, attractive, suave, cool, if the public viewed addicts as bedraggled street derelicts? Maneuvering by the tobacco industry, as early as 1905, and subsequent political pressure over the years, successfully prevented the Food and Drug Administration from having jurisdiction over tobacco—or more precisely, nicotine. It couldn't classify tobacco as a food or drug. It had no power to regulate it. So we, and the children who started to smoke after us, didn't know we would be almost instant addicts.

Now the law is changing and the FDA will soon regulate tobacco as a drug—not prohibiting it, but hopes to control advertising and marketing, at least. (I never thought I'd live to see the day.)

I'm gratified when I hear from old SmokEnder members who say generally, "Congratulations, Jackie. You told them so back in 1969, and they ridiculed and demeaned you for such an outlandish, unscientific idea . . . even though it fulfilled the textbook criteria of addiction . . ."

Now the Surgeon General has declared that nicotine is as addictive as heroin and cocaine. (But not to worry—this program makes it painless!)

It was acceptable to smoke almost anywhere back then. Even in hospitals. As a smoker (former) it was hard for me to complain about the little carts the aides would push around to patients, with candy, books, powder and perfume, *and* cigarettes. I was sympathetic to the patient and the visiting relatives who were under the stress that hospitals create; yet I was troubled by the knowledge that smoking was making them sick—or sicker. We convinced many hospitals to provide the SmokEnders program to their staff and the public, and then to create a reasonable smoking policy for patients, guests, and personnel. (The hard part was the personnel part. The professional staff rebelled most vigorously.)

Now, smoking is banned in hospitals. I still feel sorry for

those few wretched smokers who stand huddled in front of the entrances of hospitals—a mixture of all personnel: white gowns, lab coats, suits, overalls—frantically dragging on a cigarette for a quick fix. Recently I visited Johns Hopkins Hospital in Baltimore. They had a well-enforced no-smoking-on-premises policy. It was a cold, sleety February day. At each entrance to the Medical Center were little groups of people—from doctors and nurses to administrative and maintenance people—puffing away and shivering in the cold. I hope to reach as many as I can with this book or the SmokEnder program, or the audiocassette program, so they don't have to endure that indignity, *and* to steer them clear of unnecessary health problems and premature death. (Center for Disease Control reports that since 1950 almost 2.5 million people died from lung cancer. Since 87% of the deaths were caused by smoking, that means that 2,175,000 smokers died unnecessarily. If they hadn't been enticed to start smoking as youngsters, they wouldn't have gotten lung cancer! It's as simple as that.)

Smoking is now banned in some of the most unlikely places, too. For instance, the Department of Defense has banned smoking in all indoor work spaces, including military bases around the world *and* the Pentagon. That makes the world's largest office building smoke-free. I suppose foxholes are excluded, if they still fight wars from foxholes.

By 1994 the states of Maryland, Vermont, and Washington, the cities of Aspen, Colorado; San Francisco; San Jose; and New York, have banned smoking. Incredibly, the mayor of New York City (Giuliani) has ordered the Marlboro billboard removed from Shea Stadium. About 1,500 municipalities throughout the U.S. have enacted bans on smoking—most restrict smoking in virtually all public places. As I write this, the snowball of taxes and bans and social ostracism will gather tremendous momentum, so that most states will ban smoking in public places and increase tobacco taxes to cover the increase in health care costs that smoking causes. A pack will soon cost four to five dollars in the U.S.A. It's six dollars in Canada now! It *really* saves immense health care dollars, even within four to five years. (That's about how long it takes for a former smoker's body to return to that of one who never smoked—although recovery starts from day one of quitting.)

The most incredible ban, I think, is that, as of this writing, eleven baseball teams ban smoking in their stadiums; eight have special smoking sections.

Fast food chains are following suit—a money saver for them at the very least: McDonald's, Taco Bell, Jack-in-the-Box, and several others have banned smoking by employees and customers—chain-wide.

Smoking is banned in all schools that receive federal money. That means almost all public schools. Significantly, it includes faculty lounges, too. That was a stopper for us when, in the seventies, we presented SmokEnder programs for the students and were asked to recommend a smoking policy for several high schools. The faculty objected to including their lounges as non-smoking areas; the students objected to allowing faculty smoke on premises when they couldn't. Protest sprung up overnight! Even the unions became involved.

I consider this ban on smoking in schools as a gigantic move toward a smoke-free America. We can help children avoid starting to smoke by limiting their ability to smoke during school hours, at least. That reduces the chance of many becoming hooked. Chalk up another for reduced health care costs!

California and Massachusetts raised cigarette taxes by 25 cents to fund tobacco education, research, and medical service programs. Michigan followed suit and tripled their tobacco tax to 75 cents, despite a multimillion-dollar opposition by the tobacco industry. Sales of tobacco have dropped dramatically in all cases. Apparently, money is a more powerful motivator than self-preservation.

The Department of Labor announced that it intends to regulate indoor air quality by banning smoking altogether or limiting it to an enclosed separately ventilated room—in the six million workplaces regulated by the Occupational Safety and Health Administration.

One of the most indicative items: for the first time since 1930, two models of automobiles will be made without ashtrays. Chrysler broke the news, saying that only about 16% of new car buyers smoke. (They will continue to have cigarette lighters, though, for other purposes.) When one pays those big sticker prices for a new car, one hardly wants to stink it up with stale cigarette smoke.

But clearly, one of the most significant changes is the discovery (albeit belated) that secondhand smoke, also known as "sidestream smoke" and "passive smoking," is harmful to non-smokers. What a powerful force that unleashed. When research finally demonstrated what people seem to have known for years—that smoking made non-smokers ill—things changed dramatically. The social acceptability that smoking enjoyed in this century evaporated when it was learned that secondhand smoke in homes, workplaces, and indoor spaces causes cancer, increased respiratory disease, and other problems, and that young children were especially susceptible.

Smokers are now treated like pariahs.

It's becoming too hard to smoke, it's too expensive, and it's too embarrassing.

This is a good time to quit, and this book uses these new trends to support your ability to quit:

- You'll learn how peer pressure and bans can work *for* you . . .
- You'll get the psychological support you need if you're using acupuncture, hypnosis, nicotine chewing gum, or the patch . . .
- You'll more easily jettison your addiction—without or with the patch . . . and if you're hooked on the patch, you'll get help finally freeing yourself from it.
- You'll be detoxified *before* you quit, so you don't climb the walls.
- You'll learn how to avoid gaining weight when you quit . . .
- You'll find out, step by step, why you smoke and why you've had trouble quitting in the past . . . and why and how to succeed now.
- If you love someone who smokes, you'll learn how to support them instead of making them more defensive.
- You'll find ways to help children say NO to cigarettes—even if you smoke—without making NO more enticing.
- You'll be motivated to end the "love-hate" relationship you have with tobacco—cigarettes, cigars, pipes, smokeless tobacco.
- You'll discover the Four Fears that keep smokers smoking.

- And if you want to form your own self-help group for your friends, your company, or your practice, you'll find a special Teaching Guide at the back of the book.
- Best of all, you'll realize that you CAN stop smoking and enjoy the pleasure of your new freedom!

Foreword

"Jackie Rogers has a remarkable gift. She has the ability to change human behavior by a very subtle, very gentle coaxing method. And because of her own frailties she understands very well the frailties of others.

"I benefited from her ministrations in 1979 when I walked away from a thirty-year, four-pack-a-day smoking habit.

"I don't care if you find some of the material in this book too fundamental for your level of sophistication, but within each chapter are subtle nuggets—concepts—for you to consider. When, then, you get to the *"How To"* chapter, everything will be in place and have meaning, so *You Can Stop Smoking*—easily and permanently.

"So read each chapter as if your life depends on it—because it does! It worked for me."

T. George Harris,
founder and former editor-in-chief,
Psychology Today and *American Health*

A Personal Note from Jackie Rogers

This book is a result of my personal quest for freedom from my twenty-two-year smoking habit. Like most smokers, I literally tried everything, but failed.

The reason I tried so desperately to quit during those twenty-two years was not because I suffered from any smoking-related problem (other than maybe smoker's breath and some reduction in my skiing stamina), but because of my husband, Jon. When he was a young dental student he learned the hazards of smoking—to the lungs, heart, throat, mouth, and everything else it affects—during the medical portion of his training.

That was *before* we met and fell in love.

He committed himself to helping me become a non-smoker, and over the years taught me physiology and pathology as I had never learned it before.

When I sometimes complained that he was obsessed with my smoking, he would ask, "How can I stand by and watch someone I love hurt herself, disable herself, maybe even die prematurely?"

So I tried all the books and gimmicks and free clinics and psychotherapy and cessation programs and hypnosis and even nicotine lozenges called, of all things, "Life Savers." (Not related to the candy of the same name.) They almost killed me.

My failure was not that I didn't stop smoking. I did.

Often.

My failure was that I was unable to cope without a cigarette. My body and mind twisted into painful, anguished contortions and the only relief I could find was to buy, mooch or steal a cigarette.

THE CRAVING WAS INTOLERABLE. Only another smoker can know what it's like.

I FIRMLY BELIEVED I WOULD NEVER BE ABLE TO STOP SMOKING—or, if one day the doctor declared that I MUST stop, I would probably go insane or become an incompetent zombie. I also believed that if I couldn't smoke, life would be much less attractive. I remember one morning—during one of my abstinent periods—I woke up, remembered I couldn't smoke, and pulled the covers over my head, thinking, "It's not worth getting up!"

I remember another time when I was completely immobilized without my cigarettes and a friend called and asked what I was doing. "I'm sitting here NOT SMOKING is what I'm doing!" I answered, rather stridently. It wasn't long before I succumbed. The egg man came so I bummed a cigarette from him. I knew all the smokers in my life, and their brands.

The good news is: I STOPPED WANTING A CIGARETTE! I "Cut-Off" in 1968 and I haven't had a cigarette since, nor have I wanted one.

It's as if I never smoked. Not an *ex*-smoker. I am a *non*-smoker.

I'm happy to be free. Not smoking is a pleasure I want to share with everyone who is thinking of quitting.

The method that worked so magically is one I worked out for myself at the urging of my husband and family. They said, "Stop seeking experts and become one yourself." In desperation, I researched the subject of smoking, quitting, addiction (nicotine was not then considered addictive, but I felt it might be), motivation, conditioned response, oral gratification, emotional and psychological dependency—literally everything I could think of that might have a bearing on my smoking and my inability to quit.

My background in psychology together with my experience in quitting smoking, plus Jon's knowledge of physiology, pharmacology, and anatomy, were a fortunate combination. Our skills, training and experience dovetailed. Instead of a single, one-sided approach, we were able to attack the problem from various aspects. That's why it worked!

We literally took the habit apart, and as we identified each small part of the problem we created a solution for it. But, because I've never responded well to punitive methods, I forced myself to find a positive solution.

I then put it all into a gentle, step-by-step program, one that gave me plenty of time to *un*-learn and detoxify myself from the nicotine. Frankly, I was not in a hurry to suffer again.

Remember, I truly believed I could never quit. Or at least never lose the craving.

I HAVEN'T YET GOTTEN OVER MY ASTONISH-MENT AND DELIGHT AT LOSING THE COMPULSION AND CRAVING. It was as if someone had lifted a heavy load off my heart and shoulders on my "Cut-Off" day—February 1, 1968. No pain. No craziness. No self-righteous white-knuckle restraint.

I felt then—and still feel—it was a miracle of sorts. Although it was a wonderful feeling, I wasn't sure it could last. I wondered when the axe would fall. . . .

After a couple of months of being totally free of the smoking habit, I finally believed that the craving and craziness would not recur.

With the confidence that comes with truth, Jon and I decided to try to help our friends and neighbors in our hometown, Easton, Pennsylvania. That was February 18, 1969.

It worked for them just as it had for me.

With the success of our first group, we made a conscious decision to commit ourselves to helping other smokers everywhere. I had global fantasies. I knew that anyone could quit smoking and I wanted to make it available around the world. I believed that we could phase smoking out in our lifetime by making it *easy* for people to stop smoking—because I instinctively understood that the only reason adults continued to smoke was because they didn't know HOW to quit. And if it became socially unacceptable, when all the role models quit, kids wouldn't start, because it would no longer be the "grown-up" thing to do. . . .

My mind raced with ideas and plans. People said it was impossible—that smoking was too well entrenched in our culture. I argued that chewing tobacco was once a popular behavior, but it became obsolete because chewing was no longer socially acceptable; so would cigarette smoking.

Happily, Jon agreed with me, and provided the necessary financial and emotional support.

It took us a long time to come up with a name. Finally we thought of *SmokEnders*, and the rest is history.

At this writing over one million smokers have benefited from the SmokEnder program. I get wonderful cards and letters and gifts from people who Cut-Off as long ago as 1969. They remember their Cut-Off date as one of the most important dates in their lives and want to commemorate the anniversary.

There are SmokEnder chapters in many major cities in the United States, Canada, Europe, Africa, Australia and Japan. They present the six-week seminar with consistently high success rates—both at the end of the seminar and long-term.

There are now a wide variety of smoking cessation programs, including some that have tried to copy SmokEnders, but none has been able to achieve the level of success that SmokEnders has. I'm proud of that quality, and of the people involved in SmokEnders who protect it.

But because SmokEnders can't be everywhere, I have written this book to make the program available to people who can't get to a SmokEnder seminar.

If, after reading the book, you feel you would benefit from a live seminar, you might try calling local information or the toll-free information service (1-800-555-1212) and ask for the nearest SmokEnders chapter.

During the years since 1977, when I wrote the first edition, I have heard from many readers, including SmokEnder graduates (who found the book helpful as reinforcement).

They asked questions and offered suggestions to include material I didn't think of including in the first edition. I have also learned quite a bit more about smoking and compulsive/addictive behavior in the intervening years. In addition, the social aspect and cost of smoking have changed greatly since 1977. For instance, a pack of cigarettes then cost 55 cents! Nicotine has since been recognized as an addictive substance, and low tar and nicotine cigarettes, once a product limited to people with heart conditions, now dominate the market.

Secondhand Smoke, also known as passive smoking, has been found to cause thousands of lung cancer deaths a year in non-smokers. In addition, it causes severe respiratory problems especially in children. Asthmatics suffer from increased and more violent attacks. Babies have more ear problems in a smoker's home. And much more to come . . .

It's also just plain annoying to non-smokers. As a result, smoking is now socially unacceptable!

I want this book to work for you, whether you bought it for yourself or if it was given to you by someone who loves you and worries about your smoking. Like Jon, they can't be blamed for trying to prevent you from hurting yourself. (I suggest they read the chapter, ''What Do You Say to Someone You Love Who Smokes?'')

You Can Stop Smoking is a very personal book. I lived it and I believe it. I know YOU can stop smoking—and enjoy being free—just as I and over a million SmokEnders have. Here's to a lifetime of empty ashtrays.

Jacquelyn Rogers
Box #550
Easton, PA
18044–0550
March 1995

P.S. When you finish reading this book, I'd love to hear from you. You may use the questionnaire at the end of the book or just write a note to let me know how it worked for you.

J.R.

It's Not Too Late to Quit Smoking

"Stopping smoking can significantly reduce smoking related physical problems. For the typical ex-smoker, after one year, the risk of a heart attack approaches that of the person who has never smoked, and, after five to ten years, the risk of lung cancer approximates that of the person who has never smoked. The mortality ratio for former smokers who have abstained from cigarettes for ten or more years is only slightly greater than one."

Harvard Business Review
January–February 1986

1

The Miracle of the Human Mind

A habit cannot be tossed out the window. It
must be coaxed down the stairs a step at a time.

MARK TWAIN

When I was asked to write this book, I hesitated because I knew volumes have been written about smoking both in scientific literature and in the popular press. Books and articles about how to quit smoking; books and articles about the cost to the human body and to society.

But it occurred to me that no one ever talked *to* the smoker about the "bridge" between the time when he (read throughout, he or she, of course) first becomes aware of a negative aspect of smoking and the moment when he makes a conscious effort to quit.

So I'll try to cast some light on this large and frustrating national problem and at the same time give smokers some helpful insight into their own experience, in the belief that smokers *can* quit smoking—and that the act of quitting can be pleasant and give an individual a boost that can trigger off a success spiral in his life.

1

I understand so well the frustration with which health educators and the government view the efforts that have been made and the dollars that have been spent, all with such meager results.

It's exactly this frustration that causes serious people in health education to throw up their hands and say, "People just don't *want* to stop smoking; there's no point in spending any more time and effort."

I disagree with them. I'm a radical on the subject of teaching old dogs new tricks. I believe that people *can* stop smoking and that they would really *like* to stop smoking once they've changed their preconceived ideas—about smoking, about themselves, about what it means to quit. I also believe they would succeed in quitting if they had "all their ducks lined up" and approached the endeavor correctly. Not "intelligently," not "rationally." Just correctly.

There's no course in medical school that teaches doctors "Treatment for Stopping Smoking." There's been no practical approach to quitting which spells out changes in attitude and habit patterns that are necessary even to enter the quitting stage and to achieve the possibility of success.

That's why I'm writing this book. I hope that I can help you to bridge the gap between the point of discouragement and the point at which you finally, actually, take your leap into the world of freedom from smoking. And then I'll lead you to that freedom, step by step.

I'll talk about the benefits of quitting smoking as a means of achieving a sense of personal freedom and rejuvenation. I'm not promising a new life—just a chance to improve the quality of your present life. More important—because quitting is an exercise in self-improvement and self-mastery that is very tangible—I promise that when you stop smoking you'll find it much easier to reach other goals and successes.

Somehow this works because of the miracle of the human mind: the more we use it and stretch it, the better it works and the more it expands. And because if success is achieved in one area of life, it carries over. I've been through all the hard schools. I tried all the techniques that were available at the time . . . I tried and tried, and failed and failed, until I realized that it was my own mind that was holding me back, and that only my own mind could help me succeed. In the process I thought about certain insights that eventually led to my SmokEnder program.

During those discouraging and degrading twenty-two years of smoking and quitting, I wondered a great deal about smoking. What is the secret? Where's the key to the lock that has me bound to a habit from which I desperately want to be free? Is it a pleasure? Do I really enjoy it? Do I lack willpower? Can I ever be free of that horrible craving for a cigarette? How do I get out of this trap?

I suspected there was more to it than I had been told.

During my years of wonder—and my later years of studying the problem on a more scientific basis—I discovered what I had suspected: smoking wasn't just a nasty little habit. It was far more complex than we smokers had ever been told. Indeed, it was an amalgam of a vast assortment of actions, reactions, attitudes, beliefs, emotional dependence and *physiological addiction to a powerful drug*. It was similar to the circuitry of a computer.

How was I to attack this hydra of a problem? I wanted to solve the puzzle—and more important, I wanted to free myself from the nagging, mind-consuming *craving* for a cigarette. And I wanted to walk away from it with a happy, comfortable feeling of indifference to smoking.

The quest was long and hard. And interesting. With many surprises.

The first surprise was that I did it. It worked. I'm free. With *no* traces of craving, since the day I stopped—February 1, 1968.

The second surprise was that I truly *enjoy* not-smoking. It's a pleasure I hadn't anticipated. I feel physically and emotionally *free*. And I'm able to deal with day-to-day responsibilities with much more ease and control.

The third surprise was that, although nicotine is powerfully addicting, it was not difficult or painful to detoxify myself.

The fourth surprise was the discovery that the barrier to freedom was not the habit itself—which could easily be broken mechanically, as is done in the SmokEnders program—but rather the aura of personal attitudes with which we surround ourselves as smokers: what we think of ourselves, how we deal with problems, how we cope with life, how we relate to others, how we use smoking in our search for satisfaction in life, and how we lean on cigarettes to supplement our often distorted view of ourselves.

The fifth surprise was that I came to know myself a lot better. On a level that had eluded me all my adult life. I now know that my life has been put into focus. I'm comfortable with my existence. I accept myself as I am. It's my life, and I'm the boss of my life. That was a lot more than I had expected from just quitting smoking. All that I'd learned so hard is borne out by thousands of smokers who were eventually to tell me about the same suffering, the same physical and emotional weariness, the same rationalizations, the identical failures—and finally the same joyous success.

It's important to remember always that your problem is not unique. Tens of thousands who used to feel as you do now have succeeded. You can succeed, too!

From having listened to those thousands of smokers, I can say with confidence that most smokers would like to quit but don't know how to quit. There is a gigantic step that must be taken before they can approach the actual quitting. That critical step is the prequitting phase—the one prior to the actual effort. It takes certain careful preparation similar to preparation by an Olympic athlete for the big event. And most smokers, thinking it's simply a matter of willpower, are unaware of this step, so they enter the big event without any preparation. They go cold-turkey and generally fail miserably. They were not in condition.

That's what this book is all about. It's the preconditioning step you need to get yourself into gear for quitting. It leads you through that important prequitting phase necessary for success.

But I'm not going to tell you to quit smoking—or harass you with the hazards of smoking. I believe smoking is very personal. If you want to smoke, I have no right to tell you to quit. That's your business. And I assume you're well informed and know the hazards, so I won't beat a dead horse.

The secret key I was looking for was that it was necessary to understand myself first—and to accept myself as a worthwhile human being—before I could *begin* to quit. That's what I want to share with you in this book: how to get ready to quit smoking. This isn't a classic How to Quit Smoking book, but it will probably do more to help you quit than any other book or device on the market.

I'll give you step-by-step instructions and activities to teach you how to finally quit—for good.

This book will work to get you into gear—but you must work along with it. The undertaking should be fun as well as useful. At the very least you will gain some rich new insights into yourself, some new tools to cope with the problems of daily living; and perhaps best of all, you will attain a firm grasp on the kind of maturity that brings a sense of self-confidence, serenity and tranquility.

So I hope both to transmit my enthusiasm for the pleasure of not-smoking, to give you some insights into your own smoking habits, and to increase your motivation to quit to a fever pitch. After all—motivation is the powerhouse behind anything we make up our minds to do. Once our minds are convinced that we really WANT to quit—or climb Mt. Everest, or run a marathon—it's easy!

If I do no more than that, you'll benefit considerably because you'll be closer to quitting by a giant stride; if I help change your attitudes about quitting so that you really desire to take positive action and to succeed, as I believe you can, I'll be proud and gratified.

And if you've already quit smoking but want help to stay free, this book will help you with your emotional housekeeping so that you can handle stress; deal with problems; cope with life *without* reaching for a cigarette, pipe, cigar—or for that matter, candy, liquor or your fingernails. If this book provides you with reinforcement, I'll be pleased to have helped.

Most especially, this book is written to help you make a move toward a decision: either to continue to smoke without feeling out of control—or to begin your campaign to quit. And if you begin your campaign to quit, this book should help you believe in your ability to do it—with the result that you will learn to be nice to yourself. You deserve it.

And I assure you, it's worth it.

I hope you enjoy getting to know yourself—it's the best show on earth.

$$\begin{bmatrix} 2 \end{bmatrix}$$

A Day in the Life of a Smoker

Before we get started, let's get acquainted with a typical smoker. I've prepared a composite smoker from my experience with thousands of smokers—and my own history.

Meet Robert Sanderson of Cleveland. He's an attractive, successful vice-president of a large electronics concern. At 43, he can boast the usual measures of success—house, car, boat, ski lodge in Colorado. He's devoted to his wife and three children. On the down side, his wife is changing her lifestyle by returning to school and working part-time in a nearby pharmaceutical firm as a beginning lab assistant. Her work absorbs her; her attention to home and family is reduced. As a result, Bob has to attend to many family matters. Visits to the orthodontist, or to college campuses with the oldest child, have now fallen upon him. His already busy schedule has had to be rearranged to accommodate additional responsibilities. Also, his mother is becoming increasingly less able to care for herself because of Parkinson's disease, and he is distressed at leaving her alone. It's clear to him that the only real option is to have her come to Cleveland—and live with his family. But that has obvious drawbacks.

Now let's run through a day with Bob and observe how he *uses* cigarettes.

The alarm goes off, the radio goes on. Before he's fully awake, Bob reaches for a cigarette on his night table and fumbles for his lighter. This is routine since college days, so it's now an ingrained conditioned response. If he thought about it he'd say, "I can't get going without a cigarette." Translated, that reads: "My body needs a shot of nicotine to get my adrenaline going; I'm sluggish and I need help." In some cases, it also reads: "I can't face the day—so I'll call upon my friend to stave off the dangers that lie ahead." So Bob lights up and drowsily considers that day and what faces him.

Soon he's shaving, aided by the ritual of the cigarette. It seems to make the shaving easier. If he watched the ritual, he'd roar with laughter at the sight of a grown man trying to scrape whiskers off his face while juggling to keep his cigarette dry and the smoke out of his eyes—squinting and cocking his head and drying his cigarette-holding fingers. He would see himself as a clown performing a ridiculous antic. If our Bob were Betsy, it would be a similar picture—except that she'd be trying to apply her makeup and juggle a cigarette at the same time. For Betsy, the humor is in the act of doing anything with her eyes—makeup or contact lenses. It's tough when you're squinting—especially if the cigarette is dangling in your mouth because you can't put it down on the wet sink!

Now Bob is ready for breakfast, which until recently was waiting for him. Since Natalie is rushed in the morning too, Bob pitches in to find the cereal for the kids. Oops—none left. Must go to the store. How about eggs this morning, children? No, you can't have pizza for breakfast. Natalie! Why the hell can't we keep a supply of cereal in this house? . . . No, it wasn't my turn to go to the store. . . . You knew I had to go to Chicago on Tuesday. . . . Yes, I know that was the day of your finals. . . . Natalie, can't we find some kind

of housekeeper? . . . Cost be damned . . . Yes, I know
Robbie is going off to college next year and Mother will
likely come to live with us. . . . No, I don't want to keep you
from having a life of your own. . . . Here, let me get the
coffee ready while you finish making the kids' lunches. . . .
Where are my cigarettes?

And so it goes, Bob has his hands full coping with little
problems—larger problems caused by little problems—so he
reaches for a cigarette, which steadies him, or at the very
least, relieves the tension.

Translated, that reads: I'm uncomfortable. I can't deal
with this situation and it causes me to be tense. I believe
cigarettes relieve my discomfort somehow, so lighting up
will somehow cause these problems to disappear. Bob also
uses cigarettes to protect himself from problems—and perhaps as an escape valve. Really, he's creating bigger problems for himself, because the nicotine makes him more edgy
and tense. It's a matter of chemistry.

A stop in the bathroom before leaving for work. Bob
believes smoking is an aid to regularity and has convinced
himself he would become constipated if he didn't have a
cigarette while he was on the pot or just before entering the
bathroom. Another well-entrenched ritual. Of course it's not
necessary to have a cigarette in order to move one's bowels;
it's just that Bob's body has become accustomed to expecting the shock caused by nicotine to activate his digestive
tract. Once he stops smoking, his body will return to its
natural manner of housekeeping.

He grabs his coat and the grocery list and dashes to the
car. Reaching for the keys, he reaches for his cigarettes. It
has become a requirement; somehow the ignition key won't
work unless he first lights a cigarette. This is a very subtle
means of using a cigarette. It's what we call in SmokEnders
a "hidden trigger." It's one of the reasons Bob checks his
pockets on leaving the house, to be certain he has enough
cigarettes to get him and his car going. (If he used the bus or
train, he'd light a cigarette to hasten its arrival.)

In slightly more than an hour since Bob woke up he has
used five or six cigarettes: one to help him get going; one to
help him shave; one to help him get through the uncomfortable jumble of the breakfast routine; one or two with coffee;
one as an aid to regularity and one to get his car going.

Certainly all this could be called "habit"; but if you want to free yourself of the smoking problem, you'll gain by observing how you use cigarettes—so that you can change your attitude and therefore your dependence.

At the office, before he can get started, Bob lights up. Frequently, if he doesn't really like what he has to do, he lights up before getting to his desk—and stalls around doing other things until the cigarette is finished. In fact, almost anytime Bob wants to procrastinate, he lights up. It seems a very acceptable means of putting off the task at hand—and nobody can accuse him of goofing off. He uses his cigarette as a stalling device.

As he goes through his mail, he needs to think—and so he lights up again. He has come to associate his ability to "think"—concentrate—with the power of a cigarette. In fact, he is sometimes unable to "think" if he's run out of cigarettes—which convinces him that cigarettes *are* his ability to think. This is learned behavior at its starkest. Here's how to read it: Bob wants to think through a problem. Because of a well-practiced association of "sitting back and lighting up" in that situation, and also because the nicotine level soon drops in Bob's bloodstream if he doesn't light up, he would soon find himself squirming around in search of a cigarette so that he really would be unable to concentrate. It's not the cigarette which gives him the ability to concentrate, it's the lack of one that keeps him from it! (Until Bob has trained himself to recognize these situations and is no longer dependent upon nicotine, he *will* need to smoke to concentrate. Once free of the habit, he'll be able to concentrate more efficiently. Incidentally, his ability to think creatively is limited by the carbon monoxide and other gases he inhales in addition to the nicotine. They deprive the brain of oxygen.)

The phone rings. Automatically, Bob reaches for a cigarette. (Sometimes he has one already lit, resting in the ashtray, but the phone signals a cigarette, just as Dr. Pavlov's dogs learned to salivate when the bell rang signaling food. We smokers are conditioned to light up at the sight or sound or smell of certain triggers.) A tribute to our intellectual capacity: we can learn by means of repetition. Bob isn't really using a cigarette. He's just acting mindlessly.

If he's expecting a "bad news" call, he will continue to light up until it rings. In that case, he's using his cigarettes to ward off bad news and to protect himself from difficulties.

Sometimes we feel that a cigarette will make us strong and tough. So we anticipate a "bad news" call or visit with a couple of them wolfed down. This, in fact, is one of the reasons the cigarette ad with the cowboy and the horse works so well: people are afraid of appearing vulnerable and weak in the face of a stern situation. They think if they smoke cigarettes—and that brand in particular—they will seem as tough as that cowboy.

Bob goes to the Executive Committee meeting, worried about his project and the opposition of the chairman. A few cigarettes on the way with some coffee or a Coke, and another as soon as he sits down at the conference table. Whether he makes his point or not, Bob is using a lot of cigarettes to be tough and to relieve tension and discomfort. It's really a contradictory situation, of course, because toughness calls for heightened psychic tension—and calmness requires relaxed psychic tension! Bob is using his cigarettes at cross-purposes. (The truth is, he has by this time shot so much nicotine and carbon monoxide into his system, he's wound up like a mainspring—and the chances are he can be neither tough nor cool. Just jittery. In a later chapter, I'll talk about the physical effects of all these drugs and gases and the reasons they don't and can't do what the ads promise.)

If he makes his point, Bob lights up again to celebrate. If he loses his point, he lights up to soothe his bruised sensitivities. Now cigarettes are an act of reward or self-pity. Poor me, he says, in the latter case, I must do something nice for myself. I worked hard to prepare that project, the boss just doesn't appreciate me, I'll have a cigarette and make it a bit better. (This same attitude moves into and out of all our lives in varying degrees. A woman may feel sorry for herself because no one recognizes how hard she works to keep the house beautiful, or to make a splendid meal, or how she's always the last person to leave the office. A student may be disappointed in the response he receives from his teacher regarding a paper he worked hard at researching; a beautician may suffer a moment of self-pity if his client doesn't respond with a special comment of praise for the effort; and so on.) So Bob reaches for a cigarette instead of dealing with his feelings. After he has learned to live comfortably without cigarettes, he will deal with his feelings and his previous "treatment" of them.

There was another undercurrent at the meeting that had made Bob uncomfortable. He was the only one smoking. This was new. Several of the others had been heavy smokers. Now, the only smoker, he was self-conscious each time he lit up, but he was also very uncomfortable if he didn't smoke. (His friend Alex confessed he had felt the same thing in his car pool when he'd been the last smoker. The guys would make a fuss about opening the windows, choking, suggesting he could wait another twenty minutes until he was dropped off. And he was uncomfortable if he couldn't smoke during the trip. That was one of the reasons he finally quit.)

After the meeting, which was inconclusive and frustrating, Bob and Ted, who had supported his project, went to lunch to rehash. Ted was irked that Bob hadn't come fully prepared with the charts they had talked about when they had planned the presentation. Bob tried to convince Ted that he thought Ted had written the charts out of the plan, but Bob knew he was filibustering—and he recognized his "buck passing" as cover for his procrastination. With all the problems at home, he hadn't gotten around to doing the charts they'd discussed the last week, although he had known when he promised to do them that he wouldn't have enough time. Now, recognizing his own intellectual dishonesty, he squirms inside and lights up. He's using cigarettes to relieve his emotional discomfort. Their drinks come, and he automatically has another cigarette. That one is pure conditioned response. After lunch, coffee and another cigarette.

The discussion turns to bringing in Guy Baker, an engineer in the design group, to work on improving the project. Bob isn't having any of that. Guy is light-years away from understanding the approach Bob believes is essential to success in this project. Besides, though he doesn't want to admit it, Bob has been worried about Guy moving up so fast in his department. He feels threatened. So he uses another cigarette to subdue his anxiety. Ted insists on bringing Guy into the project to give it the best shot he can. "So far, Bob, you haven't been able to sell it your way!"

Bob is outraged. Another cigarette. He begins a series of arguments and excuses to defend his efforts: he could have done it right from the start if Ted had budgeted it correctly, instead of pulling out the allocation for research into the GXH system. Both men are frustrated, so their anger finds easy breeding grounds.

Many cigarettes later, Bob returns to the office to plow through his work load. His mind isn't too clear: not only is he drowsy from lunch and the drink; he's reviewing the argument in his mind and thinking of "I-should-have-saids."

As his anger wears off, self-pity begins to enter. "Ted has no idea how hard I worked to put together that presentation. He didn't say one good word about it. He just carped about what I didn't do. Just because we didn't get a positive decision today, he's sore and blaming me. Poor me. I don't deserve this abuse. . . ." And he lights up. Now Bob is using cigarettes for one of the most common uses, self-pity. Somehow, subconsciously, he thinks/we think a cigarette will salve our wounds; put a Band-Aid on our injured emotions; "make it all better."

By four-thirty, two coffee breaks later, Bob has had several more cigarettes. He's feeling weary. He must finish the report he's working on, but he needs a lift—so he lights up. And he gets a lift, all right. For a short moment. Then he sags again, and lights up again. He's using cigarettes to pick himself up physically.

Pretty soon, he's so wound up, with all that coffee and nicotine, that he feels shaky. Leaving the office, he lights up to calm himself down. He takes a deep drag on the way out and tells himself it'll relax him. Now, it appears, he's using cigarettes as a relaxant.

If Bob stopped to think, he'd be surprised at his expectations—contradictory and unreasonable. How can he reasonably expect to have something pick him up and also calm him down?

Now, life has taken a harder turn for Bob. The office manager announced that smoking won't be allowed after next month. He can either quit smoking or go outside to smoke. With his heavy workload due to personnel cutbacks, he doesn't have enough time to get his work done as it is. Going out for a smoke—a fix—is going to be more than just inconvenient.

This evening, on the way to the train, Bob stops at the friendly little bar near the station and buys two cans of beer—a trick he learned from his friend Tom, a lawyer who commutes. This way he can catch the earlier train, instead of taking time at a bar for the drink he so enjoys. And on the trip home, he can relax with a few cigarettes and a couple of beers. It would be fine, except that each night he brings home his briefcase with some work he had hoped to review on the train. So he promises himself, "I'll do it tonight after the kids go to bed, instead of watching TV."

At his station, he lights a cigarette as he walks to his car—or, if he was lucky enough to find a parking spot close to the station, he lights up as he reaches for his keys.

At home, instead of the calm orderliness he had hoped for, he is met at the sidewalk by Robbie, in his Scout uniform. Panicked. "Daddy, tonight's the Blue and Gold dinner—you promised you'd be home early—and Mommy said you'd remember to pick up the chocolate cake at Mrs. Eliason's on your way home from the station—because we promised we'd bring some dessert—all the guys bring stuff—and Mommy said she'd meet us there later after her class . . . And now we're going to be late—and Mr. Paulis says a Boy Scout shouldn't ever be late . . . and . . . and . . ."

Usually when Bob comes home from the office, at least he can kick off his shoes and take off his jacket and have a drink as he pitches in to help get dinner, help with the homework, clean up and get schedules sorted out. That usually means a cigarette with the drink before dinner. Maybe one or two more, and another during dinner; then two with coffee.

This evening, like most other evenings when he and Natalie are not entertaining or being entertained, is a frenzy of trying to get everyone and everything put back together again. Help the middle child with algebra; fix a stuck window; remember to get a button put back on a jacket; call Mother—didn't receive a letter from her this week, and forgot to send her one last week; review the reports he meant to look at on the train. Whose turn is it to pack lunches? Who put Robbie's new red sweat pants into the washer with the white things? I forgot tonight was the board meeting at the church and I promised I would be there.

In between and during the evening's comings and goings, cigarettes are used. Frustration, anger, weariness, joy, social exchanges, stalling simply from the habit of reaching for the pack because it is there!

Later in the evening, Natalie and Bob have a chance to relax together and watch TV. That's another smoking ritual perfected. It's so automatic Bob doesn't miss a moment of viewing as he reaches for the pack and matches. He lights up and returns the pack and matches to the exact spot on the chairside table for the next time. Generally he complains because "there's never anything good on TV anymore." Bored, he smokes more.

The most elaborate ritual comes at the end of the day. The last cigarette before bed is a very conscious one in Bob's routine. After a bedtime snack and cigarette, he washes and brushes his teeth, gets into bed with either David Letterman or Jay Leno, host of *The Tonight Show*, and lights up. The timing of this last cigarette is exquisite. It should be finished just as a commercial comes on, or else Bob lights up another cigarette to finish watching an act that has caught his fancy. But the last cigarette must be stubbed out just as the TV is turned off. It is almost a religious ceremony— paying respect to the God of the Night; expressing the need to formalize the close of day; a ritualistic preparation to ensure the coming of the new day. Most of us who smoke have this routine, except that some of us brush our teeth *after* the last cigarette instead of before.

So Bob turns off the lights and goes to sleep. Or maybe he goes to Natalie. If he does, he's bound to need a cigarette after sex. No one seems to know why this is a "trigger" for a cigarette for a great number of us. Perhaps, for Bob, it's a carryover from his younger days, when he was told that that was what was done.

Around two or three o'clock in the morning, Bob awak- ens; reaches for a cigarette and sleepily lights up; wanders into the bathroom, in response to what he believes has awakened him (what *really* awakened him was his need for a cigarette/nicotine fix); finishes his cigarette and returns to bed. And then he starts the whole process over again in the morning!

Are you weary and beat-up for Bob? So is he, but he won't know how much until he stops smoking.

Bob has used smoking as a propellant, a stalling device, a protection against "devils," a comfort in trying times, a lift, to calm down, to complete a pleasurable cycle, to relieve physical and social discomforts.

Throughout the book, you'll find answers to how to deal with many of those situations without cigarettes. You will benefit from the suggestions—but before you can apply them to your own situations, you must first determine how *you* use cigarettes and smoking.

HERE'S WHAT TO DO

1. Get a little pocket notebook that's easy to write in. Carry it with you everywhere. You will be asked to use it often throughout this program. It will become your bible and your support.

2. Take a quiet half hour and write your own "case history" of a typical day and figure out how YOU use cigarettes.

(Incidentally, feel free to write in this book. Underline, highlight, paper-clip pages, use Post-it notes—so you can get back to whatever gave you insight or motivation, or whatever.)

You can refer to Bob's routine; surely some of his experiences must parallel yours. Some of your own are unique.

Be honest with yourself. Write down what you really do and feel, rather than what you wish you did and felt. The notebook you'll use is your workbook—no one else should have access to it—so you should have no doubts about writing freely and openly. You're not going to be criticized or judged.

You'll be asked in later chapters to think about your feelings and thoughts about smoking.

You've seen how most of us use cigarettes. You've analyzed your own uses. If you've done a thorough job of observing and reflecting on your "connectors" to the habit, you have moved strongly toward freedom.

Some of Bob's uses are obvious and some are rather more subtle. Here's a list to compare with your list. Check the box if you *sometimes* smoke for any of the following reasons.

HOW I USE CIGARETTES

☐ To get going physically in the morning?

☐ To "ward off" threatening problems each day presents?

☒ Automatically, without realizing you're lighting up (while shaving/applying makeup; reaching for the ignition key; with coffee; using the telephone; with a drink; coming out of the theater; while typing, ironing, playing cards, for instance)?

☒ To deal with situations that cause tension/anxiety/pressure/confusion?

☒ To subdue anxiety/fears/worries/threats?

☐ To promote "regularity"?

☒ To hasten the arrival of buses or trains?

☐ To "get going" on the job?

☒ To stall, procrastinate (to "goof off" legitimately)?

☐ As an aid to concentration?

☐ To "ward off" bad news—on the phone, in person?

☒ To get tough (backbone developer) and be able to withstand difficulties?

☒ To appear tough (avoid showing weakness or vulnerability)?

☐ To stay calm under pressure (relieve psychic pressure)?

☒ To appear calm and collected?

☐ To celebrate a point won/a good score/an accomplishment?

☒ To sooth bruised sensitivities if the point is lost/for a poor score/for a missed target?

☒ To cover feelings of inadequacy?

☒ To cover feelings of social awkwardness?

☒ To relieve the emotional discomfort caused by knowing you didn't do an honest job, or make an honest effort, or tell the whole truth?

☑ To subdue rage during and after an argument?

☑ To feel solaced when abused, unrecognized or otherwise sorry for yourself?

☑ To get a physical lift when you're tired?

☑ To relax?

☑ To observe a well-practiced ritual: with drinks before dinner? with coffee after dinner? *getting home from work*

☒ To observe the TV sacrament: watch, nibble, smoke; watch, nibble, smoke . . . ?   *turning on TV*

☒ To relieve boredom?

☒ To pay respect to the God of the Night (bedtime ritual)?

☑ To fall asleep again during the night?

☐ To satisfy hunger?

☑ To gratify your mouth's need for attention?

☐ To quell an acidy feeling in your viscera?

☑ To soothe frustration?

☑ Because the pack is there?

☐ Because you think cigarettes taste good?

☐ To celebrate good news?

☑ To complete pleasurable cycles—after sex, a good meal, drinks, good friends and talk, the last run on the ski slope, sitting down to relax after working at a hobby, finishing a project?

☒ To pass time while waiting for someone, or for something to happen (appointments, car pooling, picking up someone after school or the orthodontist, waiting your turn in the doctor's office)?

☒ Because certain sounds trigger a reach for a cigarette (an old song, doorbell, telephone ring, other sounds)?

☑ Because certain odors or fragrances trigger the desire for a cigarette—the smell of a sizzling steak, beer, burning leaves, your lady's distinctive perfume (or your man's), camphor/Lysol/ammonia, chalk dust in a schoolroom, a hard-to-place aroma out of your past . . . ?

☐ Because you're restless?

☐ To keep your hands busy?

☐ To clear your sinuses?

☑ To keep awake while you're driving?

☐ To soothe a headache, cramps, pain?

☐ To start the creative juices flowing, and keep them flowing?

☐ Because everyone is hassling you to quit and you don't
   like to be pushed around?

Uses overlap and intertwine—but you surely have recognized yourself and certain smoking connections. Most of
these are learned conditions; many are easily redirected to
less bothersome and less harmful alternatives; many are
simply not true physiologically—such as "smoking calms
me down." In fact, nicotine is a stimulant; it affects your
entire system. Or you may say, "Smoking gets my creative
juices flowing." It's the opposite. Carbon monoxide in the
blood of a smoker slows down brain function!

Take comfort in the fact that all these uses are easy to
deal with—if you deal with them individually. Together,
they're overwhelming and overpowering. That's the fact
which discourages most smokers from thinking seriously
about stopping. You have to separate them out from one another.

To break cleanly and comfortably from the smoking problem (or almost any "intake" problem—overeating, excess
use of caffeine and/or alcohol and perhaps even tranquilizers), you will want to take your habit apart and deal with
each element singly.

Consider the motto "United we stand, divided we fall."
United, the complex habit you live with is as strong as
strands of wires twisted into a cable. Divided, each one is a
slender fiber that is easily cut.

Read and follow each section of this book carefully in
order to gain control over each element of your habit and
deal with it effectively. When you have all the connections
disconnected, you'll be ready.

If you have already quit or are on the nicotine patch,
or gum, follow all the instructions and complete all the
assignments and activities—except, of course, DO NOT
SMOKE! IT'S DANGEROUS TO SMOKE IF YOU'RE
ON THE PATCH.

More detailed instructions for ex-smokers and patch users
and cigar and pipe smokers will be given as we go along.

For really wonderful results, please read each chapter
carefully and do the exercises required BEFORE turning to

the "How to" section. Don't pick and choose or feel that something isn't important or doesn't apply to you.

No matter who you are and what you've accomplished in life, if you're a smoker, you must disconnect your smoking habit like any other smoker. The smoking habit isn't a reasonable, rational condition, even though you are. So put your mind and heart into this. Make it the most important thing in your life for the next six to eight weeks.

[3]

What's the Problem?

The greatest discovery of my generation is that
human beings can alter their lives by altering
their attitudes of mind.

DR. WILLIAM JAMES,
HARVARD PSYCHOLOGIST

You know that you should quit smoking, and yet you still
smoke. You're a reasonable person. So why *don't* you quit
smoking? Because smoking isn't a *reasonable* problem.

Another thing. You may have succumbed to the belief that
you don't have enough willpower to quit. Well, I have good
news for you. Assuming you have enough will to wake up
and get going each morning with reasonable regularity, and
to perform the hundreds of duties required of you each day,
you have all the willpower you need. If you counter that it's
a matter of degree, let's remind ourselves that there are
eminent doctors and judges, policemen and firemen who
have to have wills of iron and who continue to smoke against
their best interests.

What's the answer?

I discovered that the problem of quitting smoking was
more complex than just shedding a "nasty little habit," and

that it required more than willpower, or drugs or a pep talk—certainly more than plastic pacifiers and other gimmicks. Here's the clincher: You've stopped a few times, very likely—sometimes for a day or so, maybe even a couple of weeks. Sometimes you couldn't get past breakfast without a cigarette—and hundreds of times you've said to yourself before going to sleep, "Tomorrow (or soon) I'll quit smoking: I'm killing myself . . ."

When you did summon up enough emotional energy to quit, after thousands of promises—or because your next-door neighbor, a heavy smoker, learned that he had lung cancer—you quit. By whatever means you tried—and there are hundreds of possibilities—let us say, for the moment, you did quit. For a bit. But if you were the kind of smoker I was, you were very uncomfortable, obsessed with a longing for a cigarette. Soon, hours later, maybe even days or weeks, you caved in and found an excuse to start smoking again. (Or maybe you hung in and are still not smoking but are fighting with clenched teeth and white knuckles—what I call "working on gut power.")

Either way you are miserable. You may have stopped lighting up, but you haven't really changed anything about yourself. The conditions and your attitudes about smoking and about yourself are the same. Cigarettes are your trusted "old buddies"—always there when you need them, ready to make anything bearable, better.

You feel lousy without cigarettes. Since you probably don't know what it's like to be an adult non-smoker (like most smokers, you probably started to smoke in your late adolescence), you can't depend upon feeling good as a normal state without cigarettes.

Probably the biggest condition that requires real change is your attitude about the naked act of quitting. If you haven't taken this step, or you have taken it incorrectly, you're afraid of it; you think it will hurt; you believe you're unable to quit. If, by some miracle, you ever quit, you can't imagine being able to function effectively without cigarettes. You avoid the thought altogether, except for those "once-in-a-whiles" when your sense of righteousness propels you to one more resolution to quit. But see, the manner in which you approach quitting is so negative that you couldn't get close to success if you were shot through a cannon. There's a law of nature, I believe, which has been expressed in thousands of ways, certainly since Moses. It goes something like this: If you think you can't, you can't. You're licked from the start.

Though you may have tried quitting, avoided lighting up for a period, unless *all* the game pieces were in place your chances of succumbing to another cigarette were predictable. Your smoking habit was in a dormant state. It was waiting to spring to life at the first crack in your will.

So What Is the Problem?

Peter Drucker, the respected management consultant, teaches that in order to solve a problem, one must first state it. Can you state your problem? Stop, now, and reflect: What would you say the problem is that you are attempting to remedy?

If you said, "I smoke too much," I'd agree with you, but tell you that smoking too much is just a symptom of the problem.

Perhaps you said, "I try and can't quit." That's a condition. Not the problem itself.

Or, "I enjoy smoking and hate to give up something of value to me." That, dear friend, is a rationalization. (A well-used one, I might add. I used it, and almost every smoker I speak to says it earnestly.)

So what's the problem?

The problem is that smoking and quitting is like a finely woven tapestry that is more complex than a simple "do-it-yourself" approach can unravel. The problem is: YOU DON'T KNOW HOW TO QUIT. But I will lead you through the maze and help you disconnect all the connections that have you tied up in the habit. Then you will know "how" to quit—and you'll do it. Easily. Painlessly. Even joyously, although I know you can't quite believe that at this point.

Let's look at the Problem. Here's what it looks like to me, with a few examples under each:

HABITUATION	PHYSIOLOGICAL ADDICTION	PHYSICAL ENERGY
i.e.: Conditioned response; mindless lighting up.	Nicotine is one of the most powerful addicting drugs.	Smoke for a lift—but it also causes fatigue.
COMPULSION	PSYCHOLOGICAL DEPENDENCY	ORAL
You do it even when you don't want to and even though you know its harmful to you and those around you.	The crutch. Boosts self-esteem/crushes it, too. A reward; calming; soothing; eases the pain of awkwardness and vulnerability.	Your mouth gets used to all that attention.
SOCIAL	EMOTIONAL	ENVIRONMENTAL
Easier to be with people . . .	When sad, angry, joyous; when feeling sorry for yourself . . .	The ads; the pack; others who smoke . . .

It's obviously not just a nasty little habit. It's more complex than any other excess behavior in our culture. So it needs a multimodal approach rather than just a simple pill, hypnosis session, old-fashioned willpower or some form of nicotine replacement.

As you read this book, you will be given techniques to help you disconnect small parts of your smoking relationship—a little at a time. Some of the "disconnects" are very subtle. That's why it's important for you to read the whole book, in the sequence I've written it. I know you're tempted to go straight to the "How To" chapter, but in fact the whole book is laced with how-to techniques—why miss something that will help you?

Now that you are able to see the problem clearly, you want to act. BUT, before you can act, you must WANT to change. *And you must* BELIEVE *you can!*

We all have fears, but smokers bring a unique set of fears to their quitting attempts. Fear of pain, fear of failure, fear of losing something precious, fear of gaining weight . . . the list goes on and on.

Fear becomes a real block to success. If you believe you can't do something or fear doing it, your chances of succeeding are almost zero. But if you believe you can, and overcome fear so you WANT to achieve success, your chances soar. It's a matter of attitude.

Right now I want to help you take a leap of faith, regardless of your past failures in quitting. I want to assure you you *can* quit, and if you follow the instructions in this book, it won't hurt. You won't climb the walls, because you'll detoxify yourself before you quit. You needn't gain weight—if you follow the instructions and controls in the program. You won't fail because you'll get it all together BEFORE you quit. And instead of feeling that you've given up something precious, you'll feel a more precious sense of FREEDOM.

Part of that freedom is emotional—you won't feel guilty about self-destructing anymore; you won't feel disgusted with yourself because you're not in control. You won't feel embarrassed for needing to smoke around non-smokers. Instead you'll have more confidence and higher self-esteem.

The other part of the freedom is physical. You won't be living in a drugged state anymore. *You probably don't know what it's like to be an adult non-smoker*. Your natural vitality and energy has been running in low gear all these years because of nicotine. When you stop using the drug, your body returns to high gear efficiency. It's a wonderful surprise for most people—no matter how long you smoked or how old you are.

The really good news is: YOUR BODY WILL RESTORE ITSELF—RAPIDLY—when you stop smoking.

Many smokers with horrible gagging coughs report the coughing is largely gone within one week from their cut-off date. In SmokEnder meetings, the coughing and throat clearing at the first five meetings is quite noticeable. At the fifth meeting, one week after everyone has stopped smoking, there's almost no coughing or throat clearing. And people who have poor circulation come back looking pinker each week. It's amazing. A recent report in the *Wall Street Journal* states that, according to Boston University researchers, people who have stopped smoking cigarettes for two years aren't any more susceptible to heart attacks than those who have never smoked.

So, instead of giving up something of value, you'll feel you have gained something very precious. CLEAN, FRESH, HEALTHY FREEDOM.

In this book, I'll inform, motivate, lure and guide you

through the steps that must be taken, BUT you must commit yourself to this as if your life depended upon it—it probably does—you must persevere, and most especially, you must believe in yourself. You must have the courage to say, "I CAN quit smoking." Once you say, "I CAN", the next logical step is to say, "I WILL." Don't be afraid to say "I CAN"—just as the Little Engine chanted, "I think I can . . ." You will too!

PERSEVERE

NOTHING IN THE WORLD WILL TAKE THE PLACE OF PERSEVERANCE.

TALENT WILL NOT: Nothing is more common than unsuccessful people with talent.

GENIUS WILL NOT: Unrewarded genius is almost a proverb.

EDUCATION WILL NOT: The world is full of educated derelicts.

PERSISTENCE AND DETERMINATION ALONE ARE OMNIPOTENT.

Calvin Coolidge

$$\boxed{\quad 4 \quad}$$

Getting to Know Yourself

Who Are You?

Before you can take a cold, hard (but friendly) look at yourself, you must understand the need for both personal and intellectual honesty. It may be some time since you've thought about these things in terms of yourself. Here's a chance to exercise your mind and character without exposing yourself publicly.

The objective is to strip away the bull you've built up about yourself and try to get a glimpse of the real you. It's a terrific feeling, worth all the effort.

Try to look at yourself objectively: the trick is to describe yourself as if to a third person so that you are easily recognizable. You have to include vices and virtues without shame or modesty. (The notebook you use is your personal workbook; it's private. You're free to pour your heart out without fear of criticism. That's very important!)

HERE'S WHAT TO DO

Tonite:

1. **Get out your notebook**
2. Close yourself off from interruptions. Schedule a couple of hours for this, just as you would for a doctor's appointment.
3. Write the most important facts about yourself and your life. Use the Personal Résumé questionnaire, following.

Remember, the more committed you are to being free, the more you'll comply with these instructions.

First, describe your personal appearance:
  (the usual characteristics)
  Overall impression of appearance
  What do you consider to be your best physical features, and why?
  What do you consider to be your worst physical features, and why?

Now, in order to list your personal accomplishments, embarrassments, tragedies and talents, make a personal résumé.

PERSONAL RESUME

Date and place born
Elementary School:
  What do you remember as the most poignant experience— something you longed for, or treatment by the neighborhood bully, or a huge worry?
Junior high and high school:
  Describe your "popularity." Were you accepted by the gang—or were you a loner?
  In what subjects did you excel?
  Any awards received?

Were you unmercifully self-critical of your looks, behavior, grades, accomplishments?

When did you start to smoke?

Were you anxious to be independent, resisting your parents' restrictions?

Describe the exact circumstances. Include names and descriptions of your peers and elders who were party to your first experimentations with cigarettes.

What did smoking do for you, for your self-esteem? (i.e.: felt grown up, accepted, etc.)

What physical effect did it cause at first? (i.e., coughing, dizzy, sick to stomach, etc.)

College/Military service/Other interim vocations:

Dates attended   Degrees/awards, etc.

What qualifications have you as a result of any additional enterprise after high school?

Are you satisfied with the results of your efforts? Why?

Did you miss or ignore any opportunities during that period of life which you regret now? What and why?

Can you recapture or rebuild or buy any such lost opportunities?

If you could, which would you concentrate upon now, to bring you personal satisfaction?

Employment history:

(The usual listing . . .)

If you're presently employed, how did you happen to get where you are? Did the job fall on you or did you make it happen?

Is it in a field that interests you?

If not, what would interest you more?

Why aren't you engaged in that field now?

Do you have any plans to work in that direction?

Social relationships:

Who was your first date?

How old were you?

Your first love?

How old were you?

Did you/do you date seldom or frequently while in high school/college?

If seldom, was/is it really by choice?

Did you have many friends or a few?

Describe your *best* friends from childhood to the present.

Do they have anything in common?

Do you confide in them, or are you a very private person?

If you have a mate, are you satisfied with the relationship?

   If so, why?

   If not, what are the principal reasons for dissatisfaction?

   Can you do anything to repair or correct the problems?

   If so, why don't you?

If you work, what is your feeling about the majority of your business associates/co-workers?

Friendly or aloof?

   Do you consider one in particular a special friend?

      Whom?

      Why?

      Do you report to him/her or does he/she report to you?

   Do you consider anyone a particular "enemy" or impediment to your success/happiness?

      Whom?

      Why?

      Does he/she report to you or you to him/her?

      Can you do anything to improve the relationship?

      If so, why haven't you done it?

What's your experience with neighbors?

Which most friendly?

   Least friendly?

   Describe worst incident.

   Whose fault?

Family realities:

Mother: Describe her.

        What did/do you like best about her?

        Least?

        Ask and answer yourself, "Mother, I always wanted you to _____"

Father: Describe him.

        What did/do you like best about him?

        Least?

        Ask and answer yourself, "Dad, I always wanted you to _____"

Briefly describe your relationship with:

   Sister(s)

   Brother(s)

   Grandparents

   Aunts

   Uncles

   Close cousins

    Mate

    Children

        Put a plus in front of those with whom you generally have a harmonious relationship; a minus sign to indicate a dissonant relationship.

    Personal objectives:

        Quickly glance over your life and remark on the first, the most easily recalled, the most outstanding disappointment in your life. Describe it.

        What has been the greatest tragedy in your life?

        What has been the greatest success?

        What gave you the best ego satisfaction?

        What gifts/talents/qualities do you have?

        What keeps you from using them?

Now there's a good profile of you down on paper and after a lot of thinking about yourself. Look at it and see if you can get a sense of yourself. Maybe you have to convince yourself you're worth studying. Until you're convinced, let me tell you, you are. You're special. Certainly worth the investment of your time.

Let's go to the second step of this exercise.

Since you are the sum of your thoughts and experiences, you can take the results from the first exercise and place the elements on a scale to get a hook on this person you've come to take for granted. Chances are, you will be surprised at what you find—and probably pleasantly surprised. Most of us have covered ourselves with a lot of layers to hide the raw and rough spots of awkward adolescence. We had conned ourselves into believing everyone else was "cool" and sophisticated; that we could skinny by with connivances (like smoking) to make us appear more poised. And somewhere along the line of growing up, we learned to make excuses for ourselves—why we couldn't finish a job, or get an A, or be on time—or get a promotion, or a raise. It was always somebody else's fault that we didn't fulfill our responsibility. Maybe we were too smart for the task—or undereducated? Or the wrong religion? Or too rich, or poor?

What has all this got to do with quitting smoking? Well, central to quitting smoking is getting to know yourself, accepting yourself and growing up that last little bit. That means you must stop making excuses for yourself. You must learn to be intellectually honest.

Later we'll go into the typical defense/apology reactions we all use at one time or another to get us off a hot seat—when we light up a cigarette (or grab a chocolate)—but first here's an exercise to focus on the strengths and weaknesses which we call your:

REACTION PROFILE

	FRE-QUENTLY	SOME-TIMES	NEVER
1. Do you brag to others about your ability or performance when in your own mind-view you feel you don't measure up to your words?	—	✓	—
2. Do you procrastinate and then take a defensive posture, blaming someone or something for your own lack?	—	✓	—
3. Do you claim to be "expert" in some matters in which you have only a passing knowledge in order to impress someone higher up?	—	✓	—
4. Do you feel sorry for yourself because "life is hard" and "others get all the breaks"?	—	✓	—
5. Have you played the martyr to friends, relatives and coworkers in order to be the "good guy"—liked by all—because you feel somewhat unworthy and inadequate?	—	✓	—
6. And how's your Hostility Level? Do you resent the imposition on your time by others, or interference with your plans, to the degree that you'd like to "walk away from the whole thing"—or slug somebody? (Including your parents or spouse or children or job . . .)	—	✓	—
TOTAL	—	—	—

Review your answers. Three or more "Nevers" means you are really quite dishonest with yourself. Three or more "Frequentlys" says you're dishonest with others. Three or more "Sometimeses" puts you in the normal range.

Okay. That's *you*. What does it do for your smoking problem? *It fixes the first step* in your changing view of yourself—or your *changed behavior*, whichever you choose. Necessary, because you must stop making excuses for yourself. I can hear you ask, "What has that got to do with my smoking?" All the smokers I've worked with since I started SmokEnders have asked the same thing. And here's the point:

As smokers, we use the cigarette for many reasons (which we discussed earlier in the book)—but one of the principal reasons is an excuse for our inadequacy (or what we perceive to be inadequacy).

We have come to believe we must be super "cool," competent, composed in all circumstances. And we try to uphold that image at all costs; somehow, to most of us, the cigarette is used to stall, distract, interfere, impede or cushion the effect of our incompetence or inadequacy. We feel less vulnerable to the pain of embarrassment.

This view of the usefulness of the cigarette didn't just happen to us; it was branded on our minds when we were youngsters, and it is reinforced daily by the abundance of cleverly created cigarette ads. So we *use* cigarettes. If you agree with that much, let's expose the reasons to light so that we can deal with them.

HERE'S YOUR NEXT ASSIGNMENT

1. Observe yourself as you light up for the next three or more days.
2. Ask yourself, "How am I using this business of lighting up—smoking?"
3. Write your observations in your notebook.

As you light up, consider the act in a detached manner and ask yourself, "Am I *using* this device of lighting up in some way?" You will find interesting answers, if you're honest with yourself. You may discover you're avoiding answering a question or getting on with your work; you may be seeking poise in a social encounter that causes you discomfort or anxiety; or you may be simply rewarding yourself after a particularly difficult (or boring) activity.

In this book we'll discuss more specifically what each of these "uses" is and how you can deal with each without relying upon a cigarette.

So for the next three days, simply take a fresh, clear look at the possible uses. Get out your notebook, and every time you discover a new use you make of smoking, immediately write it down. That means you must carry the notebook with you at all times—if you're serious about getting to know yourself and getting a running start on quitting smoking. If you say that's inconvenient, let me remind you that you manage to carry packs of cigarettes around with you at all times—and that's mighty inconvenient, you know.

It has been said that one of the criteria of maturity is taking responsibility for your own behavior. I believe that is true—in particular in the matter of understanding the root of our "excess" use of cigarettes, food or alcohol. How does that apply to you? Think about it.

Now use the résumé you've prepared to weigh your assets and liabilities—really your strengths and weaknesses—in order to gain a glimpse of your stock in trade. This analysis will provide a silhouette of you as a person. As the book proceeds, you will be given instructions to fill in the contours so that you can come as close as possible to seeing yourself as others see you—and then determine what you should do about it.

Sir Edmund Hillary, some people say, climbed 29,000-foot Mount Everest because it was "there." Who can argue with motivation? And who can define it? But that's what makes you tick, so you'd better find out what turns you on—and why you're what you are.

Every day you're motivated to accomplish many things—get a haircut, write a letter, pay a bill, go to work, stay home from work, go on a diet, call someone who owes you money, learn to ski, play tennis, study, dig a ditch, clean a toilet, write a poem. There are not always clear relationships between any of these actions. Why do you do them?

Psychologists tell us we have only a few natural motivators: self-preservation, ego, love, money, security . . . It's a given that self-preservation should be a strong motivator—and practically all humans are highly motivated to run like the devil to protect themselves if a man-eating beast comes charging at them. So many reasonable people (who don't smoke) assume that smokers will respond naturally to the life-threatening danger caused by smoking.

HERE'S YOUR NEXT ASSIGNMENT

1. In your workbook, write at the top of a new page: My Assets.
2. Begin to list your personal assets. Not in money value, although you might like to list your home, cars, boat or whatever, but this list should contain your talents, experiences, abilities, education, position, pride items, family, friends, personal qualities you're proud of, even your pets. It's really a BRAG list. As you think of new items, jot them down. This is important for many reasons, as you will see as we go along. The longer the list, the better you'll do. Leave several pages for this.

How stunned and bewildered they are when we continue to smoke in the face of horrible warnings. I've attended scientific meetings at which the principal topic was smoking and the treatment of smoking-induced illness where I've heard men of goodwill, medically trained, utter statements of righteous indignation regarding the mass of "unappreciative fools and oafs who are unwilling to quit smoking even though they know it's dangerous and hazardous."

Well, we're not fools and oafs because we go on smoking. (Although I don't, fortunately, smoke anymore, I speak as a smoker.) They underestimate the power of the cigarette habit and the weakness of the self-preservation motive in the presence of addiction.

We smokers face many more dangers each day than the one we perceive smoking presents. We'd have to get inside a vacuum tube to avoid them. We risk our lives driving a car, riding elevators, eating, breathing, walking across the street—so, we reason, what's one more risk? Self-preservation, in the abstract, isn't quite the high-powered motivator non-smokers expect it to be. And neither is smoking quite the same manifestation of irrational behavior they assume it is. Therefore, acting rationally and stopping smoking for that reason just doesn't work for the majority of smokers.

Smoking is bad for me. Therefore, I will stop smoking. Baloney! It works in just the opposite way.

Here's what really happens. When a smoker is anxious or threatened by real or perceived danger, his first reaction is to reach for a cigarette. When the doctor tells you you're in the process of destroying your lungs or that your heart is coming loose, your most likely reaction is to reach for a cigarette. It's an ingrained defense mechanism against danger, worry, anxiety, threats, bad news—you name it. It's a comfort to an old-pro smoker who needs his faithful "old buddy" at a time like that.

What an intricate web of relationships! Unless you, a smoker, are informed about these bonds, your chances of breaking free are very slim.

So this book will help you recognize your response mechanism and give you some tricks, tools and techniques to cope—without resorting to a cigarette.

Now let's look at the rationalizations the ego provides when we evade self-preservation. We say (and we *all* seem to have invented this one ourselves, quite independently), "But I've got to die someday—of something. I might as well die happily with my cigarettes."

Another famous rationalization seems to be a piggyback to the first. "I don't necessarily believe all that cancer stuff. Really, nothing has been proved; the proofs are coincidence and not cause-and-effect, and if it were really catastrophic to smoke, the government would forbid the sale of cigarettes!" Which is another story in itself, and I'll discuss the politics of that issue in a later chapter, because, at the very least, it's as interesting as the latest nighttime soap opera.

And the third, most classic, rationalization appears, as if to tie up the whole package with a tidy little knot: we smokers proclaim, "But it won't happen to me. It'll happen to the next guy." (This is the same defense we use against auto accidents and heart attacks.)

We build rationalizations and soon we don't know what we really feel. You know now that you've got to try to strip them away and get back to the basics of you—and what you *really* want—instead of what you have tricked yourself into thinking you want. It's easy, once you have some confidence that you can gain control over this monster habit.

HERE'S YOUR NEXT TASK

It's the first stroke in gaining confidence: Begin a new list in your notebook. Head it: I'M PROUD OF THESE ACCOMPLISHMENTS.

Sure it sounds corny, but wait until you begin to see the extent of the list, and discover the quantity and quality of successes you've had in dealing with formidable and complicated problems. We have a tendency to forget accomplishments—we seem to remember our failures; but in order to build confidence, you must build on your successes. A positive spirit comes from this, and that's what's essential if you really want to chuck smoking with grace and ease.

For the next two weeks, continue to think of past successes. Write each of them in your notebook as you think of it—and elaborate somewhat, if you can. A good idea: dig out your old appointment calendars and correspondence files to aid your memory. The results will jolt you, perhaps, but that's good. What's important now is for you to get a good look at yourself from a distance.

Your list should begin to demonstrate that you *have* conquered difficulties and achieved a lot. As you correlate that with stopping smoking, you will see, in black-and-white, that you can solve problems, follow instructions, climb high mountains, win races. An expanding list will produce a renewed sense of confidence in yourself and your ability to tackle smoking.

(If you are feeling poorly about yourself and can't find *anything* to start your list—here's one:

"I learned to tie my own shoelaces!"
—which is a pretty darned complicated thing to do when you were probably only around three or four years old. Or review the résumé you compiled. You'll find many accomplishments. And one thing will lead to another.)

I could describe dozens of cases in which smokers couldn't list any successes in their lives because they were obsessed with their failure to quit smoking. They were overtaken by hopelessness. A downward spiral of failure is pretty hard to check by yourself. When you believe you can't accomplish something, you won't. When you believe you can, you are very likely to accomplish it.

I remember talking to the wife of the head of the department of thoracic surgery in a prestigious London hospital. We met at the World Conference on Smoking and Health in London, at which her husband had been lecturing on the devastation wrought by cigarette smoking and pleading with that august gathering to educate the public to prevent the suffering he witnessed daily. He was impressive. After that session, my husband and I chatted with him about Smok-Enders.

Seated in the lobby was a striking-looking woman who had just lighted a cigarette. He beckoned to her. As she approached, the doctor, with a blend of discomfort and defiance, explained that she was his wife and that he couldn't do anything with her about her smoking. He felt it was hopeless, but even so, he wanted her to meet us.

As we were being introduced, I watched the change in her expression from cordial graciousness to defensiveness when she learned we represented SmokEnders. Predictably, she began the famous liturgy of the smoker—as I had years before:

"But I enjoy smoking," she stated. "It's one of the few things I do for my own pleasure. And furthermore," she added, "I'm healthy as a tyke, so the chance of my being felled by one of Charles's dreaded diseases is improbable. Not to worry, I tell him, but he constantly begs me to swear off my simple pleasure.

"Sometimes I force him to admit that he's had patients with lung cancer who never smoked, which proves that smoking isn't the only cause of lung cancer. [This was in

1971—long before we were told that secondhand smoke causes cancer in non-smokers.] Why, this foul London air would probably cause cancer even if I quit smoking, so I might as well take my chances and die with my cigarettes."

Sound familiar?

Now let's get back to her confidence, or lack of it, and see how it leads to the development of motivation. Stand in her shoes for a moment.

Walking down the corridor to the restaurant, I asked her whether she had ever really tried to quit. It was after I had assured her that I understood how she felt, and that smoking was a very personal matter, and that I wouldn't attempt to tell her to quit. She relaxed her defenses considerably and confided to me that she had first tried to quit years before, by simply declaring that she would not consume any more cigarettes, after her husband had described the details of a particularly tragic case. The patient, an acquaintance, was the father of two young sons, one of whom attended the same school as their own son. The holder of a minor political office in their district, he was well known and well liked. He excelled in sports and was something of a local hero. He exuded good health and vitality. The time of the local marathon event was approaching when her husband, looking particularly drawn, told her that Phillip wouldn't be running the mile in that year's meet—or ever again—because he had just detected an advanced case of lung cancer. The most he could hope for was a few months.

The woman, even now, reciting the story, looked pained. "It seemed so unnecessary, and such a waste. Phillip was so vital, yet so suddenly debilitated. And then, just as suddenly, he was gone. It was terrifying.

"But the *most* terrifying aspect was that down deep inside me, I had the sense that Phillip had caused his own death, that it was self-destruction. So it was the horror of doing myself in, rather than the possibility of cancer, that caused me to vow to give up the habit."

And she described the familiar process of throwing away the pack of cigarettes on the spot, with all good intentions. She hadn't bargained for the unbelievable craving and obsessive desire for a cigarette. She couldn't concentrate on anything for very long. Her mind continually focused on the fact that she desperately wanted a cigarette. She felt cold and hot; stomach cramps alternated with nausea. Her disposition and patience hit an all-time low.

Recalling the experience now, she remarked that she was "as unprepared for the reaction as I was for labor and the delivery of my child." She commented that she had at least received something of value as a result of her labor, whereas the withdrawal experience had provided her with nothing except a loss of her self-respect.

She described how she had finally succumbed to her craving and bought a pack, which she consumed in short order. "And," she said, "right there and then I decided I'd never put myself through that agonizing, humiliating experience again."

I asked if she'd ever tried again, in spite of her pronouncement. She nodded, wearily. "Yes," she said, "Charles was at me regularly, and so from time to time I'd go through the motions of quitting. But I knew I couldn't really quit, and I dreaded the whole wretched effort. He certainly doesn't understand, and he has deliberately chosen to ignore my requests that he allow me to live my own life. He persists in reminding me that I shouldn't smoke and that it might very likely lead to serious lung problems.

"Lately we've been trying to ignore the problem, but every time he comments about my smoking, it seems to trigger me off to light up another. Seems like something perverse within me forces me to be obstinate."

I listened to her story with sadness and sympathy; it seemed so much like my own. But I had been luckier: I had a husband who had prodded me on to finding a means of freeing myself from the problem. So I clearly understood what she was feeling—and felt I could help her at least face in the right direction.

I thought about the situation and arrived at a few reasonable conclusions:

1. Her failures had destroyed her confidence in her ability to quit.
2. She feared the pain of withdrawal.

3. She hadn't the proper motivation to quit. It was obvious she was attempting to quit for her husband's sake—not for her own interest.
4. Her "rights" were being abused: since her husband had in fact ordered her to stop, her "right" to self-determination was threatened, and human nature caused her to react by defending her smoking posture.

She was defeated before she started. I suggested she try a different approach. First, I assured her, she *was* capable of quitting smoking if she could attain the three objectives necessary to overcome her mind-set.

She wanted to know what they were; but first, she wanted to know how I could be so sure she could quit smoking. I told her that from my experience with thousands of smokers—many who were much more emotionally and physically involved than she—I knew the signs which blocked success, and that when they were removed, even the most addicted smoker was freed.

She expressed a timid interest. I think she was half afraid I couldn't help her and half afraid I could.

Here are the keys I gave her (and give you!):

First, she had to believe she *could* quit.

Second, she had to find an intensely personal reason—not just pleasing her husband—for wanting to quit and convince herself there was benefit in quitting (and in not-smoking).

Third, she really had to determine that she was worth it. This book is directed toward giving you those three keys.

Making Plans, Setting Goals

Now let's make some plans and set some goals. For ideas of ways to change yourself—if you really want to—refer back to the questionnaire under "Who Are You?" In the personal-appearance section you were asked, among other things, "What do you consider to be your worst physical features?" Start with that. If your hair is too thin or too drab or unattractive, begin a list of ways to improve your hair. One might be investigating a new hairstylist. Ask people you meet who have attractive hair what they do, where they go, what they recommend for you. You'll learn a lot, because it's very likely they had some sort of problem and found a way to resolve it.

To illustrate the importance of doing something to improve your appearance to give yourself a boost, let me tell you about a SmokEnder graduate I recently met at a conference with corporate executives who were interested in providing their employees with a means for quitting smoking. They had invited me to present the SmokEnder approach because our graduate had fine things to say about the method. I hadn't seen him for about two years, and he had changed remarkably. I couldn't quite put my finger on what was different, but he had a certain bearing and presence that weren't part of my memory of him. In fact, my memory was of a rather colorless, self-effacing gentleman.

He told me about changes he had made in his life as a result of quitting smoking, lessons he'd learned from SmokEnders that had helped him take hold of his life. It had given him the confidence to change many things in his life.

He followed a similar formula for stopping smoking and for developing other personal goals. I'll try to describe that phenomenon in this book. It's easy enough to tell someone to do something and that it will produce results. You have to be an active participant in your own "conversion."

That's what Greg McPherson told me that day. "Jackie, I heard what you said, but I couldn't convince myself, first of all, that I was able to direct my own life and secondly, that I was worth it." He talked about his feelings about himself then—feelings he now sees as "self-limiters." He'd lost respect for himself because he smoked even though he felt a heavy responsibility for his three young children and realized that if anything happened to him, they'd be in bad shape. He'd become bald young, and it had caused him self-consciousness and humiliation. He had been withdrawn in social groups, even though he'd felt he had a lot to contribute and had longed to express himself. He had always felt that he could and would achieve some level of real contribution in his field, metallurgy, but during the last dozen years he had been discouraged.

"So," he told me, "I tried it your way and it worked! First I made a list of those things I liked least about myself; then I separated out the changes that were physically and intellectually unattainable, such as being six feet tall instead of five feet eight and becoming a concert pianist when in fact I have never played the piano. But making the list was revealing. I spilled out a lot of dreams and wishes I had forgotten about.

"Then I put them in order of importance to me and gave them numbers. For the next several weeks I concentrated on each item—trying to think of ways to make a transition in my life.

"After a slow start, some ideas began to come. Just as you'd said, the mind is a muscle which gets stronger as you use it, but the difficulty is getting it revved up.

"Well, I realized that one of the biggest limiters I'd been carrying in my bag of excuses was that I was bald. And it became clear that it was one of the few things I could really do something about. I had always resisted thinking about a hairpiece, because I thought it was hokey. I told myself that if God had wanted me to have hair he wouldn't have made me bald and that wearing a hairpiece was sheer affectation. But I became aware of some top guys in my company who had quietly changed their appearance, without fanfare. They had 'lost' their baldness.

"Then I remembered the SmokEnder advice to change those things you can and learn to cope with those you can't or don't choose to. So I gave a lot of thought to whether what was inside that bald head was more or less important than what was outside it—and came to some exciting conclusions. It wasn't the hair that made me do a good job—or kept me from doing it. It was my perception of myself. But more than that, it was also my consciousness of the reaction of others to me/my baldness. I perceived they were less respectful of me than of others.

"Now that I have changed, Jackie, I'm not sure whether I was correct—whether others were less respectful of me because of my baldness or because I presented the image of inferiority and they responded to that; but this much I do know: when I got my hairpiece I began to feel better about myself, and I'm having a ball. It's like a new world for me. And I know my attitude has affected my relationships with others.

"I took a little kidding at first, but people soon forgot

about it. When I met new people, they saw the confident me and responded. I've been promoted twice and expect that I'll soon be directing my own department, which is exactly where I'd like to be.

"And one day, I'll probably start going without my 'bush,' because I will have convinced myself that it's what's *in* my head that counts—not what's *on* it—and I will have developed the attitude of self-respect that comes from knowing you're good."

We all have self-limiters: we're too fat, too thin, too rich, too poor, too gauche, too smooth, too educated, not educated enough. And it's so convenient to use external conditions as excuses.

We can all grow and expand our abilities, contacts, knowledge, experience. What keeps us from trying? What makes some people take their lives in their hands and make something happen? We've got to want to make the effort to change because something excites us. That's motivation. So we all dream about something special.

In the next chapter we'll talk about what those "dreams" are and how you should rate them and sort out what you really want in life. But to conclude this mission of finding out what makes you tick . . .

HERE'S YOUR NEXT EXERCISE

1. List what you like least about yourself: appearance, manner, temperament, personality, character traits, etc. Then list some ideas of what you might be able to do to improve each.

2. Make a list of missed opportunities you now regret. Make a sub list of those you could redress: studying business law, voice training, completing a degree or working in sales instead of accounting . . .

Here's the underlying psychological principle: one reason we smoke is for satisfaction. If you'd like to reject that concept, think about those old cigarette ads which said, or implied, "They satisfy." The cigarette companies know why you smoke.

Choose one thing that excites you *and that is reasonably possible*.

Think of all the ways you could move toward that goal. Write every idea you have about it in your book. This is how you create a plan, a map for your trip. Like a good sailor, you know which port you'd like to reach, but unless you have good charts, navigational equipment and a plan, the chances of reaching that port are very poor.

For instance, let's look at the case of a woman who called me recently. After spending the last eighteen years raising her family, she wanted to go back to the business world. She had found a good job as a records clerk for an importer before she entered the SmokEnder program last year. The work was interesting, but her opportunities were limited because her French was very rusty. She realized she could move up if she could recapture her French skills. She regretted that she hadn't kept them up, because she had been a good student and had liked French in college, but she felt she was too old to do anything about it now and accepted the fact that she couldn't rise to the occasion.

Then, because she had stopped smoking, she had a burst of confidence. "If I could quit smoking, I can do almost anything," she said. (Don't we all!) And she had been told that quitting smoking should be a catalyst to other accomplishments. So she chose as her first goal after graduation from SmokEnders getting back to her French.

"I called a friend in the language department at the local university and explained what I needed. He was delighted to discuss it with me. Actually, there were many possibilities, which surprised me."

She chose a crash-course seminar that could give her enough fluency to handle the first level of the new job. Her employer was delighted that she had made an effort to improve her ability to serve the company, and he worked out a training schedule which included additional courses at company expense.

She called to thank us for giving her the confidence she had needed to turn herself on. Of course, it was her own motivation that had done the trick.

3. List your "prime motivators"—those things which

you really like to do, which you get excited about and are never too tired or too poor to do: going to the theater or a football game; having your hair cut; shopping for antiques; working out at the health club; painting; reading porno; comparing this year's sales with last year's; going out for dinner; having friends in for dinner; writing poetry or a procedures manual.

Psychologists tell us we can know the person by his past performance. You are the sum total of all your thoughts and actions to this point in your life. So if you want to know what turns you on, look at what you have done so far. Why do you pick yourself up from a sickbed to join the gang at a political rally? Is it duty—or simply that you want to be there? When you find enough of the want-to's, you'll begin to see a pattern. You will probably learn that one of the prime motivators is *your* particular thing. Is it Ego? Love? Security? Self-preservation? Money? None of these is right or wrong. They simply cause people to do remarkable and sometimes impossible things—like climbing Mt. Everest.

This exercise will help you in several ways: you'll get some insight into your real self; you'll have a better idea of which motivator will propel you toward deciding to quit smoking; it will give you some ideas of other ways to achieve satisfaction in your life. We all search for greater self-realization, because we all know instinctively there's more to us than we've had an opportunity to express so far, our undeveloped potential. Get on with it! It's your life. Make the most of it, with a plan and confidence that you can succeed.

4. **List details of "my dream look."** Plan to spend about one quiet hour this week thinking deeply about yourself.

If you could look any way you'd like, what would that be? Write it down. Describe all the aspects of that look. Head to toe. Size, weight, color, sex, type of appearance (rugged, fragile, pretty, chic, wholesome . . .)

Next check it against your appearance. What is it that makes the difference between you and your model? Why is that model more appealing to you than the way you are? Can you do something to come closer to your ideal? If you are, in your own eyes, an unsophisticated bumpkin and you want a new image, can you work out a staged transformation of your wardrobe, your hairstyle, your posture and other externals? I should caution, however, that you may be disappointed when you've changed. Or you may be pleased. But before you decide to change into somebody else, it's important to take the next step toward self-knowledge.

When you started smoking you may have wanted to emulate someone who seemed attractive. Can you recall the "look"? Is that look/style/manner similar to the one you described on the checklist above of your "dream look"?

It's important that you become extremely critical now of your inbred attitudes about what you think you want and what you really want. How important is that "look" now? What residual ideas have you from the past? Think about that—a lot. If you're still hung up on people or ideas from ten years ago, you have some more growing up to do. Pause now, and reflect.

Here's the relationship between this concept and getting around to quitting smoking: before you can throw away the crutch that made you look older, more sophisticated, "in," "cool" and all things beautiful, you've got to decide what was so damned important about looking and acting like that.

To help you focus on what you really appreciate in people, let's explore present and future models:

5. Make a list of those few people you most admire—in any and all walks of life. Think of people you know. Then scan the world to remind yourself of persons in world affairs, government, theater, medicine, law, business, society, education, art, dance, literature—anyone who has captured your admiration by his or her performance, contribution, even appearance. Next to each name, note what you admire about him or her. Study the list. It will be revealing. Then compare it with your dream model. I predict that you will be surprised. Most of us have changed. So keep up with your own tastes—and aim yourself toward your real desires, rather than the outdated ones.

This is a double task: you have to look from a smoker's point of view and from an adult's. If you started smoking for the same reasons as most of us—to be accepted by the gang and to appear more grown up more quickly—now is the time to see what you're carrying along that still works as a useful motivator. Do you still want to be accepted by "the gang"? Not likely. Do you still want to appear more grown up? Not likely. In fact, don't you really admire independence and individualism now? Don't you do some things just to be different? Perhaps the original reason for smoking is no longer useful to you? Yes, I'd say that was true of most of us.

Instead of wanting to appear more grown up, aren't you now a little concerned about your age—and how time is rushing by? Is that another reason for smoking which is no longer valid? I'd say yes to that one, too.

The next step in analyzing your relationship to cigarettes and the smoking habit is to find out where you're going now that you've broken with the past. But before you start the next chapter, please review your work requirements in this chapter, especially to get a firm grasp on your *new* model.

What Are You Going to Be When You Grow Up?

Remember how when you were a kid that question was the center of your world? Unless you are in the midst of your education or a career change of your own design, think about what you want to be doing ten years from now.

Ask yourself: Do I like what I'm doing? Is it an end in itself, or a means to an end? What would I like to do eventually? Is it in addition to what I'm doing, or instead of? Am I often bored and restless? Is it at my job or at other times? Now that I have some job experience in one or several fields under my belt, what have I learned about the kind of job, the environment, the life-style, the demands on my time, my capabilities, my weaknesses, what bores me, what excites me?

Here's what all this is getting at. Too many smokers are unhappy with their jobs. It shows up in their smoking patterns. Before arriving at their store, office or plant, they smoke a lot. When they're asked about it, it often appears that they hate getting down to the responsibility or the hassle or the conditions of their job—and they smoke to stall the inevitable or to fortify themselves.

Once aware of this, they have been helped to eliminate this excess smoking, at least. In some cases, people change their routine to avoid what they most dislike about entering the workday. One man described his solution with a great deal of jovial satisfaction. He said he had discovered he hated to walk in the front door to his office each morning because a very cranky receptionist seemed to have saved up the worst problem calls for his arrival, and she would attack him with them in rapid-fire order, along with a bit of editorializing calculated to freeze his heart in terror and panic.

"She was a dependable, efficient person," he said, "and we weren't about to dismiss her. And there were no other positions open suitable to her skills. So I had to make the best of it."

He worked out a plan, according to his SmokEnder instructions, to identify and then "repattern" any conditions that caused him to smoke excessively. "It was like playing a game of chess," he said. "I had to think of all the possibilities and risks, and find the best way to move ahead without making things worse."

Some of the options he considered were: Quit. Sneak in a back door. Come an hour and a half earlier. (She arrived an hour before the office officially opened.) Have the relief receptionist start the morning and allow the regular woman to come in later. Put in a request for a sales job instead of administration. Talk to her about the problem. Change the routine.

He decided to confront the problem face-to-face. He spoke to the woman and told her that he had a lot of important things on his mind when he came in each morning and that he wanted to unload those before he started on new ones. He asked her to collect all his calls and give them to him a half hour after he arrived.

She didn't become more gentle or more gracious, but she did as he'd asked. He had time to put his head together each morning. The mere act of walking into his office no longer mangled his spirit for the day.

There's an exciting postscript to this case. Several years later he told me he had, in fact, always wanted to get into sales, and the exercises in solving the problem of the receptionist had reminded him that one of his ambitions was to be a successful salesman. He was proud to tell me that he's now head of a sales group which deals in international commodities. He put his administrative experience together with his German and his desire to sell, and approached the vice-president in charge of international sales. After a trial period, he was given a territory, and after eighteen months he was put in charge of his group. He's a happy man, proud of himself. "I know it sounds like an exaggeration," he said, "but I really believe I was able to move ahead because I quit smoking: it gave me the knowledge of myself and the confidence I might never have achieved."

What can *you* do to live up to your potential? *You own yourself. Everything you say or do is yours.* You may make some mistakes along the way, and you may be ashamed of some of the things you've said or done. But you can often put those things aside and say, "Well, I learned something from that goof." Or, "Now it's time for me to take myself by the seat of my pants and push myself upward, instead of standing here wishing and whining about it."

First you have to decide what you want to do that you aren't doing (always within reason). Homemakers with small children may feel burdened and limited because they have little time for themselves. Business people say they are always rushed and haven't enough time to do things at home. Until we recognize what and where we are we may spend a lot of life waiting for something to happen. And while we're waiting we can do a lot of smoking . . . because somehow the two go together. See if there is evidence in your questionnaire of self-pity, for instance; or boredom.

If you really want to quit smoking, and get a bonus from it:

Here's your next exercise. Decide what you really want to do and be. Set your goals for the short term, intermediate term and long term. Take a moment to complete the chart at the end of this chapter.

Say to yourself, "Within the next year, I want to do/accomplish/gain/complete/learn/earn/lose/find/establish or otherwise achieve (whatever you dream of) in each of the following categories." Then repeat the drill, but say "Within the next five years, I want to . . ." Then, one more time, ask yourself what the pinnacle of your life should be, in each category.

It will encourage you to know that a great many successful people use this or a similar technique to plot their goals in life. You aren't bound by any contract, and you can change your mind along the way. but this much is true: the chances are very good that you will achieve most of your objectives, once you have stated them and cranked them into your dream system. You know that old baloney about "anything the mind can perceive and believe it can achieve"? Well, it's not baloney, It's true.

So think carefully. Dream and wish, and write down what you realistically hope to achieve with your life.

It's a good idea to date your entries and review the list frequently. Also, crank into your annual routine a time to recast the list—around New Year's, or your birthday, perhaps—to modify, to check off the things you've accomplished. What satisfaction! Each year you'll decide on your new goals for the short term. The fact that you will have achieved a number of your goals during the past year will inspire you to greater ambitions. There's nothing like an upward spiral. Nothing succeeds like success.

It's hard to say what we really want to do or be. There's so much to choose from. So for a starting point, begin a list of what you *don't* want to be.

6. List all your distastes in all kinds of areas of activity, including house and home, educational disciplines, tasks, sports, social experiences, ways of travel—anything that you don't like and wouldn't like to have to do as a major part of your life. Add to this list every time you observe another dislike. From the growing list, you'll soon see the nature of your interests and what excites you, and you'll be wiser in setting goals for the future.

What has all this to do with quitting smoking? Plenty. First of all, if you reduce the level of frustration in your life, you have less need to smoke, less quick-on-the-draw reaching for a cigarette when you feel sorry for yourself. Second, if your days are spent doing things that give you a sense of fulfillment and you have a genuine feeling of respect for yourself, you eliminate several causes for smoking or for resuming smoking. Wind yourself up and go.

GOAL SETTING

	Within 1 Year	Within 5 Years	Ultimate Goal
Physical (Appearance)			
Vocational (Job/Profession)			
Educational			
Social			
Financial			
Of/for family			
Sports			
Hobbies			
Of/for community			
Health			
Other			

5

Rationalizations

When I was polishing my rationalizations and trying to evade the pressures to quit smoking, I would have found comfort in the thrust of the government—and the eager cooperation of the cigarette companies—to promote low-tar/low-nicotine cigarettes. The smoker in me would quickly classify this as a "safe" cigarette. Happy day! I'd say: I always knew they'd find a way to beat the health and disease threat. And I'd close my eyes and ears a few more years.

That's really a rip-off. All that happened was that we smoked more, were exposed to more hazards, *and* the cigarette companies made more money! Here are the facts:

There can never be a "safe" material for us to inhale into our lungs in the combustible (smoky) state. It doesn't matter if it's fig leaves or orange rinds—if it's burning and produces smoke, and you inhale it, you're causing yourself problems. (And to make matters worse, if you feel "safe," you continue to smoke in the false hope that it's okay, and you put off quitting until it's too late!)

The second part of the rip-off is that, because nicotine is addictive, you must smoke *more* low-nicotine cigarettes in order to get your nicotine fix—to maintain your comfort level. For instance, if you normally smoked a pack a day of a standard nicotine brand and switched to low-tar/low-nicotine brand, you likely would need to smoke about a pack and a half a day. (Here's something to think about: if only half of the fifty million smokers in the U.S. increased their smoking by half a pack a day, and if cigarettes cost two dollars a pack, that's 25 million smokers times one dollar, or $25 million—that's MILLION—a DAY windfall to the cigarette companies.)

Here's what Columbia University psychologist Stanley Schachter says about it in the February 21, 1977, Behavior section of *Time*:

> Current low-tar/nicotine brands may be lethal. You wind up spending more, smoking more and getting far more dangerous combustion products for the same nicotine payoff as stronger cigarettes.

In an aside, Dr. Schachter observed a more serious problem as a result of the low-tar/nicotine brands. He feels it's very likely that the low-tar brands are hooking millions of teenagers. "When I was young [he was born in 1922], that first Camel or Lucky made so many kids sick that they stayed off cigarettes for good. Now so many brands are so weak that the kids don't get sick enough to stop right away. They just get hooked."

So that you may respect him not only as a scientist but also as a man who understands the problem, it is significant to know that Dr. Schachter was a chain smoker when he conducted this research.

I suspect you've discovered that your feelings and reactions to smoking are much like other smokers'. That may be a comfort to you. Your difficulties aren't unique.

One thing we share is our ability to rationalize. Oddly, we all seem to create the same rationalizations. I thought I had invented some of the expressions I used when I was defending my smoking habit until I began hearing strangers use exactly the same words. And I have since heard the same rationalizations thousands of times from the thousands of smokers with whom I come in contact.

Here are most of the **rationalizations** I've caught in the net. Which ones have you used?

First I'd like to tell you why I believe we create these "cover stories." I used to wonder about why I said things like **"Well, I've got to die of something; I might as well die happy"** when someone asked me if I realized I was killing myself. But really, what was I supposed to tell them? "Yes, I know, Mr. Jones, but I'm really a yellow-livered, weak-willed dummy with a death wish"? My ego couldn't take that kind of admission (although that was about the extent of my feeling about myself in regard to my smoking). It was hard for me to admit I was out of control. I remember one man, a stranger, who watched me fussing with a baby carriage I was adjusting—while smoking, of course. He came over and said, "I wonder if you realize how awful you look tending that little baby with a cigarette hanging out of your mouth." And he crossed the street before I could even acknowledge that he had spoken to me. I resented anyone's interference; smoking was my own business; I'd be my own conscience, thank you. Deep down, however, I knew the others were right. Therefore, I invented some more rationalizations.

So if you say, "Well, I've got to die of something . . . I might as well die happy with my cigarettes," here's something to think about. Smoking is the major cause of *premature* death. So, as rationalizations go, it sounds good—but unfortunately, the game isn't played that way. Smokers don't just up and die from cancer or emphysema or heart disease. Although cancer is swift—usually six months—and painful, the others are slow and painful. One can be a cardiac cripple or a respiratory invalid for years and years. And you won't die "happily." It'll be torture. What does the word "maimed" mean to you? It terrifies me.

But that's not fair. I am not trying to scare you into quitting. That didn't help me, and I'm convinced that it doesn't help most smokers. (It's wonderful reinforcement *after* you've quit. You can look back and say, "Whew—I'm glad I don't have to worry about that anymore!" (See Chapter 16)

There's an important point to be made about this rationalization. It's not a question of how much sooner you might die, or even of how. The point is whether you want to dull the quality of your life while you're alive. More important than dying is how you live while you are alive—*the quality of your life*. It's not a question of living longer—or dying ten years sooner. The fact is, you don't lose your life at the end: you're losing it NOW! If you're smoking at thirty, you have the same health and vitality as a person of forty; if you're forty, you're functioning like a person of fifty. It's not a matter of chance, like cancer or emphysema. It really is happening now.

Smoking has been nibbling away at your life force little by little, since the day you started. It was so gradual, you were completely unaware of it.

You know I've mentioned many times, "You don't know what it's like to be an adult non-smoker." You'll know it when you quit, because your body will restore itself quickly, and your vitality, color, and energy will return in bursts. Try it!

Here's another rationalization. It was my prize one. It went like this:

"**There's a direct correlation between my smoking and my ability to perform, produce or create.** The less I smoke, the less I can do." This seemed to be particularly true when I worked in my art studio. If I didn't smoke, I seemed just to stand around paralyzed. I now know how difficult it was for me to overcome the variety of triggers inherent in that activity. Linseed oil and turpentine were two strong odor triggers; the conditioned-response aspect was well-entrenched, since I can't remember painting and not smoking. (I'm happy to report that I very easily broke all the conditions once I was aware of them. I now have no trouble painting without smoking—except that I have very little time for it!)

I thought that was an ingenious rationalization. I've since heard it hundreds of times—all from artists and writers who have smoked and quit.

Another, probably the most used, is "**But I enjoy smok-**

ing." You may have said it yourself from time to time. What you will learn about addiction and the "relief" from self-induced discomfort should help illuminate the "enjoyment" misconception (see Chapter 6 "The Truth About . . . Addiction"). How many of the cigarettes you smoke do you enjoy? If you smoked only one or two, we could all relax. But unfortunately, if you're an average smoker, you consume about thirty cigarettes a day. That's a lot of tar, nicotine and gases for a small amount of "enjoyment."

I sometimes compare the desire to enjoy a few cigarettes with my love of pecan pie. I could enjoy a piece of pecan pie every day—maybe even two pieces a day. But I'll tell you this: I wouldn't walk a mile for it—nor would I throw a temper tantrum and get downright nasty if I couldn't have a piece when I wanted it. It's one thing to enjoy something on an I-can-take-it-or-leave-it basis. It's another to be compulsive about it.

I suggest you observe your own smoking for the next couple of days and try to establish how many cigarettes you consider enjoyable. If you feel you enjoy more than two a day, I predict you're not quite ready to quit smoking. You must be reading this because someone is pushing you to quit.

The next-most-used old saw is **"I can quit anytime I want to!"** Generally, this is from youngsters who are just starting to smoke, or from old-time smokers who usually say it as they cough their heads off. It's too bad that kids think they won't get hooked, but I can understand why. Until recently, they have never been told that nicotine is an addicting agent and that addiction to it is as demanding as any other addiction. They should be told that many alcoholics and drug addicts confess they had a harder time trying to quit smoking than quitting alcohol or drugs. We'll discuss the addictive aspect of smoking in a later chapter.

Before you become discouraged by what I say about smoking's being tougher to kick than alcohol or drugs, let me say that the process is not tough if it's spelled out for you and you're given the proper guidance. And the physical withdrawal is not as horrible as with the heavy drugs and alcohol. Nicotine is out of your system in three days.

Back to the cougher who insists he can quit anytime he wants to: when he's asked why he doesn't quit now, since he seems to have a bad cough, the response is standard: "My cough has nothing to do with cigarettes. It's a cold I've been trying to get rid of." I sympathize. How awful to expect him to admit he can't quit. The cough probably increases his anxiety about his health, and anxiety, as you know, causes increased smoking.

Here's another popular number: **"It's my only vice—the only thing I really do just for me."** The implication is that "I do so much for everyone—my family, my job, my community, everyone—I really don't get any payoff except this simple little indulgence." What you can hear if you listen carefully is "poor me." Often this is followed by "I don't spend a lot of money on drink or clothes for myself or any other extravagances." (I used this one a lot.)

And another one as well. When I was a smoker I was pleased that the raging controversy was about *whether or not* smoking caused cancer. I would argue with Jon, my husband, that he exaggerated the seriousness of the problem. And I would not consider the fact that smoking might cause many other problems for my body. Cancer was the big thing, so I'd say, "I don't believe all that scare stuff. Anyhow, **nothing has been** *proved*—I've heard and read that many times, even in the medical journals!" There are still articles like that around, and we smokers are sharp-eyed at finding them, just as we're good at sudden blindness when articles appear that offer hard evidence of diseases and damage caused by smoking.

I remember a handsome young pediatrician who went through the SmokEnder program in Hunterdon County, New Jersey, some years ago. At his graduation, he asked to say a few words about the peculiar grip smoking can have on otherwise rational people. He described his habit in reading the medical journals: if he spotted anything to do with smoking, he quickly tucked the publication on the bottom of his reading pile. He confessed he had not read one single article about smoking for six years. Up until the time his wife had joined SmokEnders several months before him, he had felt trapped. He had tried to quit many times by himself on impulse and had finally surrendered to the belief that he would probably never quit smoking. And it was too uncomfortable for him to read the facts. So he hid behind that statement that "nothing has been clinically proved yet to indicate that smoking really causes cancer."

The key word here is "clinically." It can't be proved in the way other medical tests are conducted. It is outrageous to expect that scientists would induce cancer in live human beings. So no clinical tests on humans have been done. Therefore nothing has been *clinically* proved.

But wait a minute. Some interesting clinical experiments concerning smoking have been conducted. One famous one, done with dogs that were hooked up to smoking machines and "taught" to smoke regularly, produced two significant results. First, when the dogs were unhooked from the machine, they "climbed the walls" and howled for their smoke—which proves the addictive qualities of tobacco. Second, the tests demonstrated that precancerous tissue was found in the dogs' respiratory tracts. In those dogs who were unhooked from the smoking machines the possibility of cancer was apparently reversed and the precancerous tissue reverted to normal. A significant number of dogs that were kept on the smoking machines succumbed to cancer. The experiment was conducted by one of the most renowned and respected scientists in the field, Dr. Oscar Auerbach, who was working at the Veterans Administration hospital in East Orange, New Jersey. Although this sort of evidence would convince me, it wouldn't get me to stop smoking— only to stop using that rationalization, maybe.

But let me digress to make the point right here about damage caused by smoking. We actually see thousands of smokers in our SmokEnder seminars. Many come in pale and gasping, fighting for their breath. When they graduate, having been free from smoking for two weeks, these people are breathing easily and the color has returned to their cheeks. I receive hundreds of letters from people who say their new ability to walk around the block is a miracle. It's no miracle. The lungs can't handle the overload of tar, gases and particulate matter and a bronchial impairment. When they stopped smoking, their bodies became much more efficient. It's incredible the amount of coughing we hear at our first session compared with the last. The first session sounds like a polyphonal chorus; there's hardly a moment when someone isn't coughing or clearing his throat. At the last meeting, there's only an occasional cough. Even forty-five and fifty-year smokers with coughs that seem to tear them apart discover to their amazement that the cough disappears within the first week of not smoking.

I remember a man who came to one of the first meetings in Bethlehem, Pennsylvania. He told us he was 79 years old and smoked about forty cigarettes a day, some of which he rolled himself. We asked how long he'd been smoking and he said, "Maybe forty-five years." I said, "Mr. Helms, why do you want to quit smoking? It seems to me you might not have the same concern about sickness that some others might have—and you've gone so long without a problem."

He squinted his eyes and said, "Ma'am, I want to quit smoking because of my old lady." I said that was noble, but unacceptable. We insist that smokers enter the program with a selfishly personal desire to quit, rather than doing it for their spouse or someone else.

"I've a good personal reason, all right," he said. "I'm sick and tired of hearing her laugh and taunt me every morning when I cough my guts out." He paused and then said, "If I stop smoking, my cough will get better, won't it?"

Sure enough, Mr. Helms's cough disappeared within one week after he quit smoking. And he brought his "old lady" to graduation. She wasn't so bad—but she certainly had no sympathy for all us damn fools who didn't know how to quit by ourselves and had to come to socialize to do it.

Incidentally, Mr. Helms was retired and bored. Shortly after he completed the course he dropped in to see me and announced he had gotten to think about what we said about living fully and he felt so great that he found himself a job as a watchman. He looked about twenty years younger.

Next rationalization: **"If it really did harm people, the government would prohibit smoking."**

Yes, but it would be naive to hope that the government could and would forbid the sale of cigarettes. First of all, prohibition of alcohol backfired; congresspeople have good memories of past failures. Second, the power of the tobacco lobby—the richest in the country—has kept the government powerless until recently. The revolutionary report of Surgeon General Luther Terry in 1964 was the first crack in the wall. Little by little small (but tenacious) groups, such as

GASP (Group Against Smoking Pollution), now ANR (Americans for Non-Smokers Rights) concerned with legislative matters, bans, taxes; DOCs (Doctors Ought to Care); ASH (Action on Smoking and Health) concerned with the legal aspects); and many others, each chipping away to reach legislators one way or another. And, I'm proud to include SmokEnders—which created a grass roots movement to make smoking socially unacceptable by turning out thousands of "beautiful people" to be non-smoking examples in their companies, clubs, social groups, schools, churches and practices.

Now, at last, the government is acknowledging that smoking is a serious menace to our health—and to our economy. It is estimated that if somehow there were no smokers in the U.S., health care costs would be cut in half!

Federal, state and local governments have begun banning smoking in public buildings, military bases, federal offices, restaurants and most notably, all schools! That will help reduce the supply of new smokers. Children start as early as sixth grade now—about twelve years old. By junior high they're hooked. So if they can't smoke in school, it could deter most kids. (For more about kids smoking and how to help them say no to cigarettes—even if you smoke—see Chapter 10.)

The FDA will regulate cigarettes—the manufacture, advertising and promotion. (The FDA won't prohibit the sale of cigarettes because it doesn't want to cause misery for fifty million addicts—nor create a bootlegging underworld.)

So much for the rationalization that if smoking were really bad for us, the government would forbid the sale of cigarettes, and for the one about "nothing has been proven about the relationship between smoking and cancer!" Both are useless rationalizations now.

And how about **"If I didn't smoke, I'd be very nervous."** Because of the chemical reaction, the opposite is true. (Refer to Chapter 7 "Learning to Cope . . .") In addition, when you correctly stop smoking, you walk away from a certain hysteria. Some of us exhibit it externally and some feel it only internally. But that hysteria disappears when you've stopped, and in its place comes a certain serenity, calmness.

A lot of ex-smokers tell us how calm they have felt since they stopped smoking, and many of them say, "Since I quit smoking I haven't lost my temper or my 'cool.' "

That's due not only to the elimination of the nicotine stimulant, and a concurrent decrease in caffeine intake which results when you break the cigarette-coffee stimulus-response, but also to a strong new sense of self-confidence. When you quit smoking you have done something measurable. It's not like learning to read faster or to speak more effectively in front of people. Those are matters of degree. When you quit smoking, you have done something that changes your life measurably. And you can be very proud of yourself. What's more, you did it yourself. You may attend a program to get direction, but in the final analysis, only *you* quit.

Let's go on with our rationalizations. Here's one that almost every woman has used: **"If I quit smoking, I will gain weight!"** I've long suspected this was fostered by the tobacco industry. And people's worst fears are supported by stories of people who gained tons when they quit smoking. It reminds me of all the horror stories I heard about labor and childbirth before I had our first child. Many women had felt obliged to tell me, in minute detail, all the worst. Fortunately, my obstetrician, Dr. Warner, was alert to the danger such fishwifery could cause and made me promise not to listen to anyone but him about what to expect. He trained me in Grantley Dick Reed's natural-childbirth method, and I was actively involved in each of our four deliveries—with no horror stories. Just great pleasure at being awake and in attendance at the delivery of each of our babies.

So, in like manner, the story goes out on the "wire service" from smoker to smoker that a condition of stopping smoking is gaining weight. It simply isn't true. There's not some mystical force that connects a circuit in your system to cigarettes and that, when disconnected, causes a weight gain. I didn't gain when I finally stopped. I held my same weight for about six years after I stopped, with no thought of diet or restrictions. Now, in my advancing years, and my more sedentary life as a business executive, I *have* put on some weight. But it was certainly not a result of quitting smoking. And my story isn't unique.

When I had tried quitting prior to following the method I spell out in this book, I had tried to substitute anything I could put into my mouth, and I would gain weight. Fast. I'd have the lovely excuse I was looking for to start again. "Heavens," I'd say, "I'd rather die from a lung disease than from obesity." Of course people gain weight if, when they quit smoking, they start stuffing their mouths with everything that isn't nailed down. If I tell you that you should satisfy your mouth's need for oral satisfaction, you must understand that it shouldn't be with the wrong kind of food. You could chew on ginger root or a clove, or some other non-habit-forming item. Best of all, a routine of vigorous tooth brushing and rinsing with a pungent mouthwash after each meal and before bedtime does a great job of satisfying the mouth's hungers. It's better not to start with gum or candy, which would only give you another habit to deal with later on—and maybe cavities to boot.

Some people experience a change in their metabolism. Which is great. Your body becomes much more efficient and utilizes food more efficiently. Some people need less food than formerly—or they need more exertion to burn up the same amount of food intake. Fortunately, when you stop smoking and have more energy and vitality, you will want to do more physical things—increase the amount of time you spend on the courts, or begin swimming again, or take to walking briskly. It's more inviting now that you don't start coughing the moment you breathe deeply.

The question of weight is in your hands. If you want an excuse to start smoking again, allow the fat to build up. But remember, *you'd have to weigh about 125 pounds over your present weight to do as much damage to your heart as you do by smoking only one pack of cigarettes a day*. And when you quit smoking you can do almost anything, so losing weight is a good next goal. (If you're really concerned about weight gain, follow the "How To" steps carefully.)

Here's another old one: **"What good is quitting? I inhale more junk in the air because of all the pollution. A little more won't make much difference!"** That's an easy balloon to shoot down. Try this test. Take a clean white handkerchief and walk out into the most polluted area you can think of. Take a deep breath. Hold the handkerchief in front of your mouth and blow out through the handkerchief. Now, light a cigarette, and take a deep drag. Before exhaling, place the handkerchief in front of your mouth again, and blow through it. The black spot of "tar" from your cigarette will demonstrate to you the matter of dilution and filtration. Polluted air, although it's not pure and healthful, is much more diluted than "straight smoke" from your cigarette. There's no contest. You really don't have to go to all this trouble. If you smoke filter tips, tear one apart after you've smoked it and examine the gook that's collected in the filter. And that's only part of it. The rest is still in your lungs.

How about this one? **"I smoke because it tastes good."** Yes, I eat pecan pie because it tastes good—but by golly, if I ate twenty or thirty pieces of pecan pie a day, I'd vomit from here to Hackensack. We've already explored enjoyment and you have observed yourself smoking and found just how many and which cigarettes give you pleasure. Later you will do the same for taste and see how many cigarettes—*no, how many puffs*—taste good to you. You'll be surprised.

And what about the mornings after, when you've smoked a lot of cigarettes at a party or a meeting? I remember smoking cigarettes that tasted foul, and I remember mornings when my mouth tasted like the bottom of a birdcage. I can't tell you what things taste like to you and what you consider a good taste. You are examining your smoking conditions with a high degree of personal honesty. I expect your answer to how many puffs taste good each day will fall in the same range with the answers of our regular SmokEnders who search for taste. Frequently *none* has tasted good.

If you're getting more eager to quit smoking, I suggest you do something to change the conditions in your mouth regarding taste. Milk isn't generally considered a good partner for a cigarette; it doesn't enhance the taste of cigarettes. Find things that are opposed in relation to your taste for a cigarette. Avoid the "ham-and-eggs" combinations, such as coffee and a cigarette. End your meals and snacks with something that doesn't naturally lead to a cigarette.

The importance of this exercise is to give you some awareness of your ability to control your smoking "environment." Once you realize you can interfere with many of the conditions of smoking in rather pleasant ways, you will look forward to quitting as a hopeful challenge rather than a hopeless battle.

"**It's my buddy!**" This is a pet rationalization of most smokers—and for good reason. Cigarette ads direct their message to this concept to a large degree. They know we have developed a close relationship with our cigarettes and our brand. A major advertising campaign once touted "Me and my ———"—the implication being that a smoker and his "buddy" could lick the world alone and he didn't need any other (human) relationship. I don't know whether it sold cigarettes, but it imprinted the idea strongly in a lot more minds. (I discuss the effect of cigarette ads in Chapter 8.)

If you're anxious to "disconnect" yourself from another subtle connection to the habit, examine your "friendship" toward your cigarettes and your brand. Ask, "What kind of friend would 'control' me—and perhaps cripple or kill me?" Begin to change your view of Old Buddy to *a friend who betrayed me*. If that's still too strong for you, think of it as an old flame from your youth, someone in whom you lost interest who chases you and who coaxes you to return.

This thinking should lead you to the best possible attitude after you quit smoking. Indifference! *You should not feel that you've given up something precious, but simply that you've lost interest in smoking*.

And "**I can't imagine myself not smoking. It's part of me.**" This is probably the only valid statement in the lot: most of us started so young we don't know what it's like to be an adult non-smoker. We have no idea what capability an undrugged adult body has, in endurance, energy or sustained good health. Nor our minds. We can't really know how much we limit our thinking processes because we don't know what our full capability is.

I was impressed with the observations of a former smoker who received his doctorate from MIT many years ago and has been highly successful in his field. He wrote to me about a year after he had quit smoking, "I have discovered that I labored under about a 25% handicap while I was smoking; now, having quit smoking and dealing with the same theoretical and practical problems, I realize that I am able to comprehend, reason and calculate much more clearly and rapidly. I regret the years spent working at less than my fullest capacity."

And this is true of *cigar and pipe smokers*, too: the same effect of carbon monoxide upon the brain which reduces peak performance. Because it doesn't matter what you smoke—cigars, pipes, high- or low-tar cigarettes, lettuce leaves, cellulose or shoe leather. They all produce carbon monoxide as an end product of combustion. As you draw in the smoke, you subject yourself to substantial doses of carbon monoxide. There's no way to escape it.

That brings up another form of rationalization. Pipe and cigar smokers often say, **"I'm safe because I don't inhale."** Or **"Cigars and pipe smoking aren't harmful—it's cigarettes that do the damage."** Unfortunately, both statements are cover-ups. Pipe and cigar smokers, when reading this book, should translate the word "cigarette" to "pipe" or "cigar," because all I have said about cigarette smokers applies to cigar and pipe smoking too. In fact, cigar and pipe smokers use smoking in additional ways to insulate themselves—and they have an exceedingly strong view of themselves as smokers. It seems a great part of their person. Truly a physical extension of themselves.

Okay, smoking seems to be part of you. There's nothing else you do with such frequency. Nothing. And your mental image of yourself is as a smoker. You picture yourself attached to a cigarette just as you picture yourself with a nose attached to your face. That's what must change. You must be able to see yourself without a cigarette before you can begin to disconnect from the habit.

ANOTHER ASSIGNMENT: Imagine yourself as a non-smoker. In your mind's eye, see yourself "clean"—without a cigarette in your hand or in an ashtray near you. Observe people you admire who don't smoke, and begin to model your mental image of yourself along their lines. Begin to look forward to a time when cigarettes don't dominate your existence; when you can come and go anywhere, anytime, without considering whether you have enough cigarettes, if you'll be permitted to smoke, if you'll offend anyone; and especially when you can say to yourself, "I'm no longer controlled by that tube of chopped-up vegetables wrapped in paper; I am my own person."

Visualize yourself as a free person.

6

The Truth About Physical Addiction and Psychological Dependency

One remark common to all smokers is: "But I enjoy smoking." Almost every smoker has said it. It's hardly surprising. Not only is it bound up in your right to choose how you live, but the implication is that you deserve some simple pleasures in life, and if smoking gives you pleasure, you don't have to deprive yourself of it. (You bet I understand. I made that remark thousands of times.)

Since nicotine is addictive—which means the body requires that a certain level of nicotine must be maintained in your bloodstream—you become uncomfortable when you've gone beyond your normal time for another dose. Usually you react by reaching automatically for another cigarette. It takes only seven seconds for the kick to reach your brain, so you've quickly added another shot of nicotine and all's well.

Let's think of the times when you've run out of cigarettes. Perhaps it was Sunday morning, after you had had a gang over the night before. After the initial panic, and after you've hunted the house for a hidden pack, and been reduced to retrieving butts, you become aware of some strong physical signals from your body. At first, the vague discomfort in your gut becomes a kind of twitchy uneasiness. Soon you start feeling sweaty, cranky, maybe headachy, downright mean. Although you've probably promised yourself you'd finish dressing, have breakfast and do some routine chores before going to the store for cigarettes, you find yourself driving or running to the store, grabbing a pack, wolfing down the first drag and feeling some sense of peace again. "Ah, that's better. I really *enjoy* smoking. What a pleasure!"

What happened was that you were damned uncomfortable without a cigarette because of the lowered level of nicotine in your bloodstream. *Lighting up relieved your discomfort, and you translated that to mean "enjoyed."* This concept was a real breakthrough for me. I call it the Discomfort Theory.

Here's what to do for the next three days:

1. **Observe your sensations of discomfort** during those times you're forced to do without a cigarette past time for your dose. (Yes, dose. You need a "dose" of nicotine to maintain your comfort level just as a diabetic needs his insulin—except that when you stop smoking, the body becomes accustomed to doing without the nicotine and you can be comfortable without any additional doses.)

2. **List your sensations** as they occur and note the amount of time between each sensation and a new one. A good list could easily run to about fifteen items.

(If you have already quit, or are on a nicotine replacement, you'll need to disconnect the "enjoyment" connector; think about those times when you climbed the walls until you could get another cigarette.) Here are a few entries to help you get started:

Gnawing in the pit of the stomach.
Tightness in the throat, a sense of thickening.
Sweaty palms, leading to chills, later perspiration.
Rapid pulse.
Sharply increasing respiration.

Inability to concentrate on anything other than getting another cigarette.

Now you have got hold of a big secret: nicotine is addictive—and you are addicted. If you can accept that, the rest is easy; the rest of the problem is manageable. It's not a matter of changing your character by willpower. I remember the relief I felt when I discovered this. In the old days, the popular belief was that cigarette smoking was "habituative," that nicotine didn't meet the criteria of addiction. (Smoking was just a nasty little habit.)

Even Dr. Luther Terry's famous Surgeon General's 1964 report, in which he linked smoking to cancer for the first time, did not acknowledge that cigarettes were addictive. That concept was purposefully rejected in connection with cigarettes.

It was not until the Surgeon General's 1988 report that cigarettes were deemed to be addictive.

How cruel. So many have died unnecessarily. Painfully. Prematurely. They didn't know they'd be addicted when they took their first cigarette around fifteen or sixteen years old. And then they didn't know how to quit. (A recent survey indicates that 70% of kids who smoke would like to quit but can't.)

The question of addiction was ridiculous. It came as no surprise to smokers that cigarettes are addictive. Most smokers who had tried to quit would say, "I'm hooked!" They knew. Then when Congress recently challenged the tobacco industry to admit that nicotine was addictive so the FDA could finally regulate this highly addictive and toxic drug, most smokers were surprised to learn that it hadn't been classified as addictive years ago.

Back to 1968, when I was focused on getting free of my stubborn 22-year, two-pack-a-day habit. I asked my husband, Jon, a dentist, "Does nicotine meet the criteria of addiction?" He opened his textbook, the bible of the pharmacologists, *The Pharmacological Basis of Therapeutics*, by Drs. Louis S. Goodman and Alfred Gilman, and it was clear that I was addicted.

1. Tolerance for the drug. The need for more and more of the drug to satisfy a craving. Yes. I had to smoke as much

and as regularly as my body had become used to or I'd develop withdrawal symptoms. I'd climb the walls. (What a perfect expression for that feeling.) And I didn't know any smokers who ever smoked less, over time. Each of my smoking buddies were up to two or more packs a day. Yet we all started with just a few a day. Then, little by little, we increased the number of cigarettes we smoked each day. We were lucky. Our tolerance to the drug, nicotine, was relatively low. I've worked with people who needed four and a half to five packs a day to satisfy their nicotine habit. (Happily, most quit nicely!)

2. Measurable physical withdrawal symptoms. During my research, I tested myself by going without cigarettes for several miserable days. With the help of my husband, who is knowledgeable about such things and obtained the necessary equipment, we measured everything we could. Yes, I had measurable physical withdrawal symptoms (and some awful non-measurable psychological symptoms, which I'll discuss in later chapters).

My body temperature dropped. My respiration and pulse rate slowed. Blood pressure lowered. I perspired more. I felt tingles in my fingers and toes, and got drowsy, constipated, thirsty, salt-hungry, chest pains, bleeding gums, and more. (These were later catalogued and used in the program as "Symptoms of Recovery.")

3. Dependence. How difficult it is for the user to quit in spite of the evidence that it causes physical harm?

I tried to quit for 22 years with no success, in spite of the fact that my husband had clearly demonstrated to me the harm I was doing to my body by smoking. Over the years, he patiently described the systems of the body and how they are affected by nicotine, tar, particulate matter physiology and the resultant pathology. I was quite convinced that my insides were a black and rotten mess—the anxiety of which only made me smoke more! After the Surgeon General made his horrifying report in 1964, the harm I was doing to myself was confirmed, and yet I continued to smoke—although I tried harder to quit.

So, deciding that cigarettes were indeed addictive, I built my program on that thesis. I felt that since I wasn't heroic, I must figure out a way to detoxify myself gently and slowly so I wouldn't suffer those physical withdrawal conditions. I reasoned that if I could tame the addictive part, I could concentrate on the psychological dependency—the social, oral, emotional, and conditioning aspects I had identified earlier.

Making that decision was a major turning point. And it worked. I quit without any further craving. It was a wonderful freedom. I felt I had been given a magnificent gift, and I wanted to share it with smokers everywhere. So I founded SmokEnders and vowed to take it to the moon, if there were smokers there. (So far SmokEnders has only gotten as far as Tasmania, but I haven't given up.) The reason for this book is to reach as many as possible, and so far it's working. I receive wonderful letters from people who write of their "amazing" success.

Why, I wondered, could I as a smoker recognize the condition as an addiction while the scientific and health community eschewed the designation? The health agencies feared that to label smoking as an "addiction" would put it on the same level with heroin and imply equally severe detoxification suffering, which would so intimidate smokers that they'd be unable to quit. Years later I realized the truth. Cigarette companies are adamantly against having cigarettes (nicotine) declared addictive for several reasons. First, because it creates a negative image for their product. An "addict" calls up the image of a derelict in most minds. Second, if it became public knowledge, many beginning smokers (children under fourteen) wouldn't start. Third, if a person is addicted, he or she no longer has the choice to stop using cigarettes simply by choosing to not smoke anymore. And that opens the cigarette companies up to liability suits. Fourth, as an addictive drug, nicotine would be regulated by the FDA—a disaster for the tobacco industry (more on that elsewhere).

Here's an example of addiction at its worst. There is a disease, called Buerger's disease, which affects the circulation. The blood vessels that supply the extremities become constricted each time nicotine is inhaled. This can lead to gangrene. But the condition can reverse itself completely if the nicotine intake is completely cut off.

I remember a particularly moving incident some years

ago. I was working late at the office when the phone rang. It isn't unusual for me to receive calls from smokers late at night asking for information about quitting. They take action impulsively when they get sufficiently disgusted with the habit. I expected the usual "I'm fed up with smoking; I just burned my blanket. How do I go about joining SmokEnders?" This woman was crying. She begged me to help her husband. Right away. Here's what she told me:

"Jim and I have been married for about twelve years. We moved to this area so we could buy a little photography shop and have a country life for our children. We have three. Two boys, thirteen and eleven, and a girl, nine. Jim is the photographer. A good one. I do some photography, order materials and I'm the bookkeeper. We make a living and have been getting along okay. Then, last year, Jim got gangrene in his left hand. The doctor told him it would help if he quit smoking, but Jim didn't quit. He doctored for the hand, but it was no good. It hurt terrible. And it smelled fierce. He couldn't work, so I took over that too. And then the doctor told him he had to cut off his hand. So this year I've been helping Jim while he learned how to work with only his right hand."

She had trouble talking, because she was sobbing and trying to control herself.

"Then," she continued, "Jim began having trouble with one of the fingers on his right hand. He put off going to the doctor because he was scared, I guess. By the time he told me about the sore, it looked terrible. We went to the doctor, and he said, 'Jim, you must stop smoking or I'll have to remove this finger and maybe even the hand!' and Jim said, 'How much time do I have to quit, Doc?' And the doctor said, 'I can't give you more than five days, Jim.'

"So we went home and I pleaded with Jim to quit. He's only thirty-two and so wonderful and healthy otherwise. I guess I worked on his nerves, because he got angry with me and told me it was his life and he'd do what he wanted with it.

"I think he tried to quit for a day or so, because there weren't any cigarettes around one day. But yesterday, he was smoking again. I didn't know what to say or do. Today he's smoking just like always. When I asked him what we were going to do for a living if he had no hands, he said, and this is what made me crazy, 'That's not what worries me. I'm worried about how I'm going to smoke with no hands!'

"And tomorrow's the fifth day. Please, can you help him to stop smoking right away! I just saw your name in the newspaper."

So this is what experts and doctors see. They see the emphysema patient who can't breathe without a machine at regular intervals who puffs away on cigarettes in between; the heart-attack victim who knows his system has difficulty even in an oxygen tent and who starts smoking first chance he gets.

Why haven't doctors routinely told their patients to quit smoking, especially before the onset of disease caused by smoking? Let's have a little charity for the medical and dental professions. In the past, most physicians and dentists were convinced that smoking was detrimental to their patients' health. They learned in their pathology and physiology courses that nicotine was a lethal poison; commercial uses are pesticides, poisons and as a tanning agent on leather and hides (not to mention what it does to your face); that it constricted the blood vessels so quickly and sharply as to cause a decrease in circulation which could be measured by a drop of up to 4°F or more in skin temperature; that the effects of the constriction last from twenty to forty-five minutes after even one cigarette (American Heart Association); that in some cases circulation was so impaired as to cause Buerger's disease. Buerger's disease is called "smoker's disease" because it's so uncommon in non-smokers. They also recognized that patients with bronchial afflictions suffered more serious and prolonged seizures if they smoked. It didn't take a lot of scientific study to observe that smokers with respiratory ailments coughed wildly with each puff of smoke into lungs already working hard to deal with minimal breathing.

Dentists, too, were aware of the increased difficulty smokers endure. They saw the harm smoking does in their patients—the diseased and flabby gums, the stained teeth and foul mouth odor, the precancerous lesions and horrifying cancers of the tongue, lips, cheeks and any other soft tissues of the oral cavity.

For a long time, they took a strong and honorable position: insist that the patient cease smoking immediately "or else." This was a little more difficult for the doctor who was a smoker, since the patient could make the observation that apparently the doctor himself wasn't thoroughly convinced.

But the bigger problem arose when the patient left the doctor's office, vowing to quit, but found he was unable to deal with the problem without help. He climbed the walls. He was obsessed by the desire for a cigarette and he couldn't concentrate on anything else. He became wild and disagreeable, and so he returned to his doctor and said something like "Doc, I'd sure like to follow your instructions and quit smoking, but somehow I can't manage to do it without help. Give me a pill or something to help me."

Is there a pill for quitting smoking? There is not. If the doctor prescribed a nicotine substitute (lobeline sulfate/ Nikoban) or Nicorette, a nicotine-based chewing gum, or now the nicotine patch, patients soon found that they needed much more to help them than that; if the doctor prescribed a tranquilizer, the patient relaxed so nicely he lost his resolve to quit and had a pleasant "I don't give a damn" attitude in its stead.

If the doctor was inclined to help by counseling, the patient required frequent appointments and undisturbed time, which was not only very costly but often ineffective, since medical and dental schools do not offer courses in "Breaking the Smoking Habit." (They have, of course, many courses in what to do about diseases that result from smoking.) So we addicts had very little to go on but our own instincts, judgment and conscientiousness.

My physician, a smoker, advised me to schedule appointments with a psychiatrist (then at $25 an hour) when I pleaded for help in quitting smoking. Unfortunately, he was a smoker too and counseled me to "cut down." He felt my husband had a problem because he was so upset about my smoking.

The doctors learned that commanding a patient to stop smoking produced instant frustration, because the patient would quickly respond, "Okay, Doctor, but *how* should I quit? I've tried many times and I can't." The doctor had nothing to offer, so many doctors understandably skirted the issue. They'd often say, "Well, keep it in moderation." I asked my doctor, "What do you consider a moderate amount?" and he replied, "Oh, around a pack or so." I was happy about that for a while, because I had conned myself into believing that I smoked only a pack or so. (Really it was more like two packs a day, but I never kept a record and my purchases were very irregular, so I fooled myself for years.)

If you would like to have your doctor supervise your quitting, with the help of this book, I suggest you discuss it with him. Write for a "Facilitator's Guide"; see "A Final Note From Jackie" in back of the book for information.

You'll see, as we progress through this book, how important the concept of addiction is to your success. For instance, we discussed one of your pet rationalizations, "If I didn't smoke, I'd be very nervous and tense"; now you can recognize clearly the effect of the drug on your system and you'll be comforted to know you can function more effectively without it.

Let's look at the concern of the health agencies in regard to addiction. First, there's the matter of degree of addiction. Certainly, opium and heroin are much more powerful than nicotine.* Increasing doses of heroin/opium per day are required to cause the desired effect. The body is more profoundly involved physically. Heartbeat and breathing rates are dramatically changed, while nicotine affects the bodily systems less violently. So the tortures of withdrawal, as depicted in movies and novels about the drug addict, are not nearly as bad for the smoker. But it can cause a smoker a fair amount of distress if he goes cold-turkey. And it's one of the reasons you've probably avoided quitting, even avoided thinking about quitting. Each time you tried, you were probably miserable and you succumbed to a cigarette. And now all you can remember is the misery.

That's reasonable. Who likes to suffer? (This is an interesting spiral: the thought of suffering as a result of quitting strengthens your belief that you enjoy smoking. Quitting

---

* As far as addiction is concerned, opium and heroin are far more intense and create a greater effect upon the mind and body; however, nicotine is a more potent poison. One drop in the eye of a rabbit kills it within seconds.

could be a no-win situation. But it's not, as you'll discover within the book.)

Here's an important fact, which should give you much support when you're ready to quit: nicotine is out of your bloodstream within three days after you stop smoking. (Unless you're very sedentary or bedridden.) Think about that. Three days and you're no longer craving the drug.

It's quite possible that you might have succeeded in quitting smoking during a previous attempt if you'd known that. Getting past the third day is a giant step toward success.

Knowing that addiction is one of the obstacles to success, you can face up to it. It's not some vague bond that keeps you chained to cigarettes. They contain a powerful drug, and it's better to know what you're working against.

Base your notions on stopping smoking on the fact that nicotine is addictive and that you can deal with the addiction in solid, tangible terms. I'll tell you how later in the book— when you're fully prepared to act.

To sum up the arguments toward freeing yourself from the habit, remember that nicotine is addictive, and its absence causes discomfort; lighting up is simply a relief of a self-induced discomfort.

Nicotine is poison. Can you ever again say, "But I *enjoy* smoking"? Say instead, "I can do without for three days; then I'll soon be free of the habit."

And indeed, you soon will be free.

Alas, the addictive component is only ONE part of the problem. The *psychological dependence* is the other component with which you must deal. That's why, even if you once quit for more than three days, you started smoking again. That's why nicotine gum and patch usually don't work alone.

The next chapter begins to dissolve the psychological dependence, and Chapters 14 and 15 will eradicate it completely. But please don't turn to those chapters until you've lined up all your ducks by reading each chapter in order. And as strange as it sounds, I want you to keep on smoking until you are properly prepared to quit in the final chapter of this book.

Note: If you are presently using Nicorette or a nicotine patch, you are addressing only the chemical (addiction) portion of the habit; the psychological aspect of your habit, discussed in this book, will be invaluable to you. (In the SmokEnder program, we don't use any nicotine substitute or replacement for "weaning" the smoker. Instead, we have a unique technique which detoxifies smokers by getting the nicotine out of their blood stream BEFORE they stop smoking. In that way, they don't climb the walls or lose control, and quitting becomes an exciting and positive event rather than a painful one.)

Unless you're on the patch or other nicotine replacement:

CONTINUE TO SMOKE WHILE READING THIS BOOK SO YOU'RE FULLY PREPARED TO QUIT.

7

Learning to Cope with Stress—Without Cigarettes

(For a Treat Instead of a Treatment)

How did we get this way—dealing with a hundred tasks, responsibilities and problems, like a juggler in the circus? How can we take on so much responsibility for others when we can hardly deal with our own problems?

It's the same for all of us, and it adds up to the same thing. Tension. Hysteria. Pressure. Short tempers. Guilt. Hostility. More cigarettes . . . *But do cigarettes really make anything better?* That's one of the key concepts of the SmokEnder program which all members usually see clearly at the end, whether or not they agreed with it when they entered the program. *Cigarettes don't make anything better!*

In this chapter, I will demonstrate to you that you can cope more effectively and less hysterically *without* cigarettes—and that smoking may, indeed, be one of the *causes* of your poor management of some situations. We'll explore some of the reasons why we rely on cigarettes to solve our problems. And we'll take the new you along to try on both your old and new attitudes toward the things you deal with every day. Life has an unbelievable way of dealing out sharply agonizing pain and anguish—and sometimes simultaneously, magnificent joy and happiness.

Do you ever wonder how some people stand up under misery and torment? I often think of Mrs. Rose Kennedy and wonder how she kept her head together through her lifetime of extremely sad experiences. For most of us, a retarded child is the ultimate in sadness and heartache; Mrs. Kennedy had a retarded child. To lose an eldest son is heartbreaking; Mrs. Kennedy lost her eldest in the war. She lost her daughter Kathleen in a plane crash. Say that the law of compensation balances such sadness, and three of her sons gained prominence in national affairs. One became President, one Attorney General and later a senator, and the third also became a senator. How could she endure having two sons assassinated? Any one of us must empathize and know we'd have difficulty enduring the agony of lost dreams and promise as well as the pain of losing loved ones. How can Mrs. Kennedy have coped with all this? Her husband had been rendered helpless by a stroke, so that she could not rely upon him for solace. It seems unbearable.

I puzzled about this for years, because I doubt that I could have withstood a quarter of the emotional trauma without coming apart and losing my senses. I read an interview once in which a journalist asked, "Mrs. Kennedy, we have all wondered how you have been able to cope with the events in your life so courageously." And she responded, "It isn't the events in your life that matter—it's *how you respond* to the events that matters." Mrs. Kennedy learned to cope.

You can cope too, but let's look at some tricks and techniques that can be more helpful than a cigarette.

Sorting It Out

The best way to gain control of your hassles and worries is to put them into tangible form. Then you can deal in a direct, businesslike way—instead of feeling that you have a thousand worries, problems, responsibilities. Here's one trick that is borrowed from the best of business management.

PREPARE A BUG LIST

List everything that's worrying you—or bugging you. When you've finished your Training to Cope with the help of this book, you should have formed the habit of writing a Bug List for yourself at least once a week, so you can get the accumulation of problems off your chest and get on with taking care of some of the things you can deal with. What really happens is that you put priorities on problems and deal with the most important first. You will also see that some things are really not so serious, some things will repair themselves without any attention (somehow some problems just dry up and blow away if you ignore them) and some of the bugs are just "supposin' " worries.

Earl Nightingale, the famous motivational expert, said that 80% of the things we worry about never happen, 15% we can't do anything about, so we really have only 5% to deal with—and that's not too awesome. Why worry?

Let's find the 5%. There's a sample list on page 80. Make your own in your notebook and add to it during the week. As you take action on or eliminate an item, draw a line through it. It feels good to have wiped out a worry visibly. And it helps in the future, when you look back and see some of the things you were worried about. It can be almost funny.

But that's a lesson for you, too. You can train yourself not to clutter your head with unnecessary worries and problems. You have to state a problem before you can solve it. And writing it in this form forces you to put it into a concise statement. Then you can write some meaningful alternatives from which you can choose your best action. Then you can act.

That brings us to the next condition you should examine in your campaign to restyle your life in order to reduce the need to smoke: anxiety.

Anxiety

Anxiety is defined as a "painful uneasiness of mind over an impending or anticipated ill." That's Webster. The garden-

Sample Bug List

RANK (Importance)	ITEM	ACTION NEEDED
#3	Prepare report for Monday	Find 3 hours alone; ask Charlie to discuss best approach; borrow a computer.
7	Visit Aunt Tillie in hospital	Call her to tell her we're thinking of her—will come on Wed. nite.
1	Tuition for State College	Rearrange payment schedule of mortgage, student loans, grants? Try for a loan? Suggest Sis get a part-time job?
5	Mother-in-law lives with us; very little privacy now.	Consider redoing Sis's room as a private studio-type room with a little kitchen for Mother; she needs privacy too.
2	Our anniversary next week! What, when to get a gift and do something about it?	Call the Simmonses, ask them to join us for a day in the country to celebrate; or tickets to the concert? Buy a card to send on Tuesday!
4	That cough is getting worse.	Appointment with Dr. Franklin; consider quitting smoking . . .
6	Promised to give a talk next month. Scared; uncomfortable about it.	Decide to do it and get to work learning everything I can about the subject; or decide not to do it and call the chairman today. Get it off my mind.

variety definition is fear and self-doubt over something you can't do anything about, frequently something you can't even state. (When you know what's bothering you, either do something about it or worry *constructively*. Learn from it.)

Charlie A., a junior in college, is tense about an economics exam. He's done as much as he can to master the material, but he worries about whether he can get a top grade. For a few days he allows himself a vague sense of impending doom and is helpless to do anything about it. On Sunday night, the night he prepares his Bug List, he has to state the problem. What he discovers is that his problem isn't vague at all: he hadn't given himself enough time to study the material to get his A. Now he has to develop some alternatives and act on them. The anxiety is reduced, just as a swollen ankle is, in direct proportion to the firmness applied to it. Charlie has several alternatives. He can withdraw temporarily from the student orchestra and free himself for some extra study time; he can spend the weekend at school studying, instead of visiting his girl; he can cut down on his preparation for his other subjects which is risky; or can resign himself to less than an A.

Charlie chooses from among the alternatives what he perceives as the best solution. It may be the wrong one, but at least he got off dead center and did something to move his case along and relieve his anxieties.

There are two things to think about. The anxiety alone could cause him to fail in the exam; anxiety seems to paralyze us. Also, life is filled with the necessity to make decisions, and the wisest among us realize that we will "win a few, lose a few"—nobody's perfect. How hard are you on yourself? Do you expect always to have the right answer; do the right thing; make the right decision? You need an escape valve.

1. Ask, "Why has this task got to be done?" You may find that you'd been plodding along from habit with a project, using a procedure that is no longer useful.

2. Promise you'll examine your attitudes about tasks you set for yourself. Set the goal realistically. Remind yourself that this is an imperfect world.

Once the goal is set, go to it. If you go beyond your goal, that's terrific, but not necessary.

3. "Is there a better way to do it?" Often we inherit obsolete practices and never stop to reexamine the procedure.

4. Do the very best you can.

President Carter, in his first "chat" with the American people shortly after his inauguration, pledged to "Do the best I can," and, he added, "I'll make some-mistakes . . ." To be comfortable with yourself, you must be honest with yourself. Do the best you can.

When we start making excuses for our behavior, we get into emotional trouble and smoke more. How often do you hear someone say, "Well, I didn't know you wanted that today." That's one example of the kind of "excuse" that puts us down in our own eyes.

To sum up, here's how to deal with anxiety and frustration and reduce your need to smoke:

1. Ask: Why is this really necessary? If you find it isn't, give it a low priority on your Bug List.
2. Ask: What is to be accomplished? Set a realistic goal. State what should happen, by when, to what degree (or in what amount), at what cost in time and money.
3. Ask: Is there a better way to do it? Faster, shorter, pleasanter, cleaner, cheaper . . .
4. Do it! And do the best you can.
5. If you're a perfectionist, give yourself permission to make mistakes.

Stress

Many smokers feel that they can't quit because their lives are so stressful and that smoking puts them on an "even keel." It's not surprising that we feel that way. We've been told that smoking steadies our nerves.

I used that excuse too, and whenever I did without my cigarettes for a couple of hours or days, I became an animal. So, I reasoned, cigarettes keep me calm.

But it isn't quite like that. I was unprepared to "do without" my dose of nicotine and my "old buddy." I felt physically rotten and emotionally deprived. I was angry with myself and everyone in the world for having had this dirty trick played on me.

I'm delighted to assure you it doesn't have to be like that. You will be emotionally and physically prepared for the time when you choose to quit—and you will do it with a smile on your face. Another bonus: You'll be *calmer* when you quit because your body won't be jarred chemically into a hyper-mode each time you light up. For a fuller explanation, read on.

Our Bodies

How can a stimulant act to calm us down? I'd like to describe another scene in the average smoker's routine. When Jeremy wakes up, he reaches for a cigarette to get himself going. What gets him going? Nicotine.

Smoking a cigarette introduces nicotine into the system via the soft tissues of the mouth as well as through the lungs. The body reacts violently, since nicotine is a poison. The reaction causes a flow of adrenaline and other hormones which bring us to a higher alertness and give us (briefly) increased energy in a crisis by elevating our blood-sugar level. This causes a momentary "lift"; it is followed, however, by a burst of insulin which causes a sharp drop in blood sugar after the "danger" is past, and the result is a feeling of fatigue. Fatigue causes anxiety, self-pity, low-grade dissatisfaction and general discomfort—which, for a smoker, are signals to reach for a cigarette to get a lift.

Consider the fact that you repeat this process twenty, thirty or forty times a day and for however many years you have smoked. (I repeated it about forty times a day for twenty-two years.)

If you could see inside your body—as in the old Alka-Seltzer ads—you'd see a lot of action. In addition to glands squirting adrenaline, your pancreas is busily dealing with the glycogen your liver is shooting. All this produces a temporary rise in your blood pressure, which increases your heartbeat rate by at least nine beats per minute (a smoker's heart beats around 10,000 extra beats per day), and all that activity apparently influences the levels of fats circulating in the bloodstream. Yet another reason why smoking causes heart attacks.

At the same time, the red blood cells are obstructed from

their mission of carrying oxygen to the heart and brain because of the carbon monoxide and other gases in the cigarette smoke. In fact, "as much as 20% of the blood pushed around by the heart of the smoker is not working so far as carrying oxygen is concerned. Since the heart has the highest oxygen requirement per unit weight of any tissue, any change in the supply of oxygen could affect the heart first, and thereby increase the risk of an attack for the smoker."*

This marvelous machine, the body, has an additional mechanism working to stabilize these ups and downs— another law of nature at work: "To every action there is an equal and opposite reaction." Indeed, after this swift high, the body, in its attempt to maintain itself at a constant level (known as homeostasis), drops into a depressed state— below the level of comfort—as it replenishes the supply of hormones, enzymes and sugars that have just been expended in combat. You feel blah. It's not imaginary.

So Jerry reaches for something to give him another lift. This time he reaches for coffee.

Coffee is also a stimulant, as you know: it, too, constricts the blood vessels and starts the heart pounding and the blood pressure zooming. The lift can be so potent, you shake. "Coffee nerves" aren't imaginary. On the way to work Jerry has two more cigarettes, and around ten o'clock begins to think about a break for coffee. As we know, blood sugar needs to be maintained at a certain level for comfort. If one has too much, he has diabetes; if too little, hypoglycemia. Most of us have a properly functioning system, but when we burn up more sugar than we have in reserve because of increased emotional or physical demand we feel weak, or woozy, or lightheaded. Dr. Alton Ochsner, in his book *Smoking and Health,* referred to this condition as the "Blind Staggers." If you have it, you know what he meant. He found that smoking causes the level of blood sugar to drop. When your blood-sugar level is low, you certainly look for a lift—but a cigarette isn't able to boost you up high

*William Likoff, M.D., Bernard Segal, M.D., and Lawrence Galton, *Your Heart* (Philadelphia: Lippincott, 1972), p. 175.

enough, so you go for coffee, and the combination of the caffeine and the nicotine does the job. So Jerry can work until lunchtime. Lunch is something like a hamburger, french fries and coffee or Coke—and a couple of cigarettes. About three o'clock Jerry becomes weak and twitchy again. So he has another coffee or a Coke, or iced tea—it's the same shot of caffeine and sugar—with a couple of cigarettes.

By now Jerry is so hyped up he can't sustain his energy level very long, and he may start chewing on candy or, if it's available, drink some beer or other alcohol. His body is begging for sugar and he responds to it. And like nicotine and caffeine, I believe sugar is also addicting. The more you use, the more you want; when you stop for a week, you lose the craving. Try it. It works!

He gets home really tired; has dinner after a drink or two; smokes; has some more coffee very likely; smokes; watches TV or goes out for the evening; smokes; drinks coffee, beer or liquor; comes home; has a snack and some more coffee and a final cigarette.

In the morning he wonders why he feels tired. It's because he's drugged and worn out. His body has never had a chance to build up reserve resources; he constantly overdraws his account in his energy bank. It's not hard to understand why smokers' hearts give way sooner than those of non-smokers.

"Well," you say, "what should Jerry do instead of running in that rat race he's caught in? In fact, what should *I* do?" Because, very likely you're caught in it too.

Since fatigue heightens anxiety and self-pity, and makes it more difficult to cope with stress, the best way to treat fatigue is to *prevent* it! Fatigue is most often caused by insufficient rest, improper nutrition, poor circulation, emotional depression or drugs, such as nicotine, caffeine, and alcohol.

Obviously it's easier to quit smoking if your mind and body are in the best possible condition.

The following steps will prepare you in every way for your big "event," just as Olympic athletes prepare for their big events.

BE GOOD TO YOURSELF

Treat yourself with the greatest possible respect—as you would a very important person. After all, you are the most important person in your life! Be willing to rearrange your priorities as you would for your best friend. *Put yourself and your personal needs first for the next four to six weeks.*

Think of it this way: if you were seriously ill and the doctors advised you that the only way you could recover was to participate in an elaborate and time-consuming series of treatments over the course of two months or so, would you hesitate to follow their instructions? Of course not. You'd rearrange your schedule and make it a top priority. I don't want to overdramatize this, but your quitting smoking is a serious matter—perhaps the single most important thing you can do for yourself at this stage in your life. Wherever I go, I meet SmokEnder graduates who tell me the same thing, "I quit smoking x number of years ago and it was the best thing I ever did for myself!"

So the prescription to put yourself and your personal needs first is a serious one. Here are some steps to take.

Write these topics and instructions in your notebook:

1. REPATTERN. Examine your daily routine. Don't do things because you have always done them that way. If certain routines are frustrating or unproductive, jettison them. In the book *One Minute for Myself,* Spencer Johnson suggests you ask yourself, "What's the best way to take care of myself?" and then be quiet for a minute and think. The answer will come.

2. LET GO OF THE TRIVIA IN YOUR LIFE. If something isn't personally satisfying, say, "Sorry, I don't have time in my schedule just now. Maybe another time." Then plan to do something wonderfully satisfying for yourself. This is when you will refer to your "Rewards" list. (For more ideas, refer to the "Rewards" list in back of the book.) Don't feel guilty about taking care of yourself and don't be a martyr. Doctor's orders!

3. FIND TIME FOR PHYSICAL ACTIVITIES—which make you feel great, as well as being a weight control measure—at the start of each day plan ahead to do one thing to get your circulation going. (I'll give you some good ideas further on.) Remember, without robust circulation, the billions of cells that comprise your body are malnourished.

4. NOURISH YOURSELF. A few simple guidelines from my research for DietEnders, my weight wellness program, can help you avoid putting on weight, while keeping you in top condition. Remember, we don't recommend you try to *lose* weight during your quitting experience. Do only one thing at a time. It's too much to expect of your body and mind to change two important behaviors at once. The good news is that when you conquer one behavior it's easier to tackle another. We call that the "ripple effect."

How often have you said—"If I can quit smoking, I can do anything!" It's true—within limits, of course.

• **Avoid simple carbohydrates.** All sugar, including white table sugar, brown sugar, honey, turbinado, etc. This includes sugar in your coffee, plus all the pastries, cookies, and candies that contain sugar. It's not just because sugar is fattening—the bigger reason is because sugar excites your insulin which, in an attempt to maintain homeostasis, overshoots and causes a sharp drop in your glucose (blood sugar) level. When that happens, you feel weak, weary, and a sort of hollow hungerlike feeling. And when smokers feel weak, weary, or hungry, they reach for a cigarette to give them a lift. (When it happens to dieters, they reach for sweets.) So avoid sugar as much as possible for the next several weeks. Incidentally, you'll get a bonus: by avoiding sugar, your energy rebounds naturally, and you'll have more prolonged vitality than you've had in a long time.

The good news is there's one sugar that doesn't excite your insulin: fructose. Biochemically it is absorbed differently than all the other sugars. Instead of being absorbed quickly into your bloodstream, it proceeds to your liver and resides there as glycogen until your body calls for glucose, at which point the glycogen is converted into glucose and slowly flows into your bloodstream—never exciting your insulin! I am grateful to Jeanne Jones, noted food authority, diet author and consultant to the American Diabetic Association, for bringing this subtle but important fact to my attention. It is still a poorly understood aspect, but a well-documented fact, that although fructose—a natural sugar found in fruits and corn—ultimately converts into glucose just like all other sugars, it doesn't activate the insulin process.

Understandably, you might reason that eating an orange—or other fruit—would be useful since they contain fructose. Unfortunately, they contain other "oses"—sugars, to which the body reacts with a burst of insulin. And in a short time you may become weak and weary and have that hungry feeling again. Certainly, if you're concerned about weight after you quit smoking, I suggest you don't reach for a fruit or fruit juice as a pickup UNLESS you have had a high protein meal to counterbalance it.

In this program, you may use a small amount of grapefruit or orange juice as a pickup instead of a cigarette, when you determine that you need a lift. However, fructose would be a better choice.

Recently, a process has been developed to produce fructose in tablet form. I have tested and used the tablets successfully, both for a lift and to preload before a big meal so I don't get overhungry. They work wonderfully.

Unfortunately, the tablets have become difficult to obtain. I am trying to have them formulated and made available for my program, but until I do, you might want to use granulated fructose, which is available in three-gram packets in most grocery stores. Melt a half packet (about one-half teaspoonful) on your tongue (surprisingly not sickeningly sweet), or add to a cold beverage, or sprinkle on cold cereal. Fructose doesn't work in hot foods.

Carry some packets with you. (A tip: they attract moisture, so carry them in an airtight Ziplock or vial—or, if you ever used a cigarette case, use that.) Use "as needed" when you need a lift or when you're hungry, instead of a cigarette. Up to ten half packets a day is okay for now. You'll use less and less after you quit and your body stabilizes—unless you want to use it as an aid to weight loss.

Other uses will be discussed in later sections.

Note: According to Jeanne Jones, diabetics should treat fructose as an exchange, or ask the doctor for direction.

If you'd like me to inform you when and where fructose tablets become available, see page 240.

• **Increase complex carbohydrates.** Fruits, vegetables, grains, seeds, nuts, dried peas, beans and lentils—we can eat a lot more starch and still lose weight. Avoid white flour, but otherwise enjoy whole grain, semolina pasta, great ethnic foods like red beans and rice, tacos and beans, bean, barley and rice soup, and other good combinations. Keep an eye on how much fat, grease or oil you use. Your body needs some, but if you want to control your weight, cutting down on fats will give you faster results.

• **Include protein at each meal.** Current thinking is that Americans eat more protein than they need. I disagree. Based upon my own personal experience *and* from my experience working with thousands of smokers and dieters, I believe adequate protein plus *sufficient* complex carbohydrates (vegetables, grains, seeds, dried peas, beans, legumes), *modest* amount of fruits and juices, and some fats are necessary to maintain energy, reduce hunger pangs/fatigue, and control weight. What is "sufficient"? For my needs, the protein must exceed the carbohydrate. During my bout with Chronic Fatigue Syndrome for several years, I learned that I did not metabolize carbohydrates efficiently. I not only became more fatigued, but I also gained weight. When, then, I increased the protein intake, and reduced the carbos, my energy returned, I lost weight—and my lipid profile and blood pressure improved considerably.

Of course, if you have a lipid problem, you will want to discuss diet with your doctor. Even so, I recommend you consider this approach. You may be skeptical, but let me remind you how quickly "conventional wisdom" changes—and how contradictory each "new" finding is. For instance, for a while, margarine was "better" for you than butter; then, oops, it's not good for you. Butter is better.

But for the purposes of your project to quit smoking, to the extent that you must be in the best physical condition possible, I would strongly encourage you to increase your protein, relative to your complex carbohydrates. Obviously it would be wonderful if you could also avoid simple carbohydrates: sugars in any form except fructose.

The point is this: if you don't "fuel" yourself adequately, you lose energy—feel tired and/or hungry—either of which makes you reach for a cigarette.

What protein? Poultry, fish, meat, eggs, and dairy products. If you're concerned about weight, avoid fatty meats, skin on poultry, excess cheese (which is high in sodium and can be constipating.)

If you'd like more information about the higher protein diet, I recommend a book, *Dr. Atkins New Diet Revolution*, by Robert Atkins, M.D., a cardiologist who became frustrated with seeing his patients relapse shortly after successful heart surgery. He determined there needed to be a lifestyle change and a changed nutritional approach. It's controversial, but it worked for me.

• **Eat a good breakfast.** Get your energy going right from the start. One reason most smokers have a coffee break and smoke more around eleven in the morning is because they have run out of fuel. Breakfast for most smokers is usually a cup of coffee or two and a few cigarettes.

I stopped eating breakfast when I was in junior high school! It took too much time, I hated oatmeal, my older friend in high school said she didn't eat breakfast anymore so I rebelled. I have a hunch a lot of us went that route. But now we must assess our patterns. Breakfast is very important. If you were a car, how far would you get if your owner didn't fill your tank but asked you to travel on empty—on the promise that fuel would come "later"?

You might do it, but it wouldn't be efficient, would it? Of course not.

When I finally took breakfast seriously, I realized I had to have something that would be nourishing, quick and easy, something that was not fattening, delicious *and* portable, since I'm often on the road. So I created a formula of all the necessary ingredients—seeds, nuts and grains—put it in a plastic storage bag and carried it with me. Over the years, I've adjusted the formula until it is in perfect balance. It provides me with a complete, delicious meal. Perfect for breakfast—my family loves it, too. I also use it for a quick lunch or mid afternoon or bedtime snack. Lots to eat; great fiber, it's filling, sticks to the ribs for hours, and is satisfying: chewy and crunchy.

I've registered the name: Meal-In-A-Bag®, and hope to be able to make it available soon. If you'd like more information, see page 240.

Until then, I suggest you make a mixture of good cereals and seeds. Some good-tasting, reasonably healthy cereals are uncooked oatmeal, Shredded Wheat, and Grape Nuts. Beware of those that declare they're healthy but contain several kinds of sugars. Good seeds, which contain essential oils, are sunflower and pumpkin seeds, for instance. Make a mixture and pack a half cup or so in a Ziplock bag, to carry with you for "emergency" meals and "serious snacks." That's what we call them in DietEnders.

• **Consider eating four to six small meals a day,** instead of two to three larger ones. This is a fine weight-control device, as well as a means of eliminating fatigue. For example, have breakfast at seven, mini-meal at ten, lunch around one, mini-meal around four, dinner at seven, mini-meal at ten.

Listen to your body: eat *when* you get hungry—don't wait until you're overhungry. You won't eat more than your body can handle. You won't be logy and sleepy after such meals. Each regular meal will become smaller because the Serious Snacks will have reduced your appetite.

A Serious Snack should consist of a whole grain, some protein, and perhaps a vegetable. Some ideas:

A glass of non-fat milk and ½ banana
A slice of chicken or turkey on whole wheat bread with a little
    mustard or horseradish, and some crunchy raw vegetable
A small chef's salad
A "Meal-In-A-Bag"® with milk
Peanut butter on whole wheat bread (a complete protein)

Incidentally, be careful about the brand of peanut butter; most have hydrogenated fats and dextrose, and precious little peanut butter. Smuckers is good and generally available nationally. Or have the peanut butter ground to order, if possible.

• **Take vitamins.** During this time of preparing to quit smoking—and in fact, during your entire life—you must give your body whatever it needs to prosper. Vitamins, minerals, enzymes, and trace elements are all necessary to life; some come only from the food we eat. The body can't manufacture the raw materials internally. It depends upon you to provide the missing elements. If you provide high-quality nutrients, your body functions best—and you feel good. If you provide low-quality nutrients, you feel poorly, and your body breaks down.

Doctors have told us that if we eat a well balanced diet we will get all the vitamins, minerals, trace elements and enzymes we need. I wish that were so. My own study of thousands of DietEnders weekly intake charts show that even nutritionally conscious people are unable to obtain all nutrients needed. And if they get close, the poisons and chemicals in the air, water and food processing destroy much of the vitamins they consume.

For instance, nicotine destroys vitamin C, so although you may be drinking lots of orange juice, your body is probably starved of vitamin C.

I recommend you take a good vitamin supplement during the preparation-to-quit phase and for some time after you quit.

The best—and by far the easiest—way I know to get ALL the nutrients one needs is with a product my family has been using for more than fifteen years. It's called ALL-1 (formerly TRN), a powder made by an ethical company, Nutritech, in California. I simply put one scoop in a shaker or jar with some grapefruit juice, shake it, and drink it. It's not unpleasant-tasting, either. That's all I need for the day. It contains all the vitamins—in correct proportion to each other, minerals, enzymes, trace elements (very necessary for smokers), and all the essential amino acids . . . the protein our bodies don't make.

Sure beats trying to figure out which minerals work with which, and how much of each vitamin is enough or too much. Instead of an assortment of jars and bottles of capsules and tablets, it's all in one. (That's why it's called ALL-1, I guess.)

In fact, because it contains protein, it can be used as a complete meal—instead of breakfast, for instance, as a weight control.

I'm a true believer in vitamin supplementation. Science is beginning to demonstrate that we benefit greatly from a variety of vitamins—to prevent cancer and other diseases, to maintain good health and to improve our immune systems.

So now that you're quitting smoking, you will want to do everything possible to be in great condition; not just to repair the damage you might have done so far.

I urge you to look into taking a good, complete vitamin

preparation such as ALL-1. If you want more information about ALL-1, or to try it, call 800-235-5727, Ext. 95.

If you want to try to find a complete tablet or capsule, be careful of those that seem to be able to squeeze everything in one small tablet. They're unlikely to be *complete*. Also, test one tablet in a glass of water to see if it dissolves—and if so, if it does so within a few minutes. If it doesn't disintegrate quickly, it's not dissolving in your stomach—so you're not getting the benefit you need.

There are only a few products I feel worthy of my recommendations, and ALL-1 is one of them.

• **Reduce caffeine and alcohol.** When you follow the directions for quitting at the end of this book, you'll automatically reduce the amount of caffeine (coffee, cola, tea) you drink—without feeling deprived. It's important that you cut down on caffeine because it is a powerful central nervous system stimulant. In other words—it jangles your nerves. And when you're hyper, you smoke more to calm yourself down. Right? (Wrong. It doesn't!)

Alcohol acts to depress the nervous system and nicotine is a stimulant, so when you quit smoking, alcohol will have a greater depressant effect. In addition, alcohol dulls your motivational intensity. When you need all your powers of determination and concentration, you can't afford the ''what-the-hell'' attitude that liquor provides.

So for now, when you have choices, choose to drink juice, milk, Postum, decaffeinated coffee, caffeine- and sugar-free colas, instant bouillon, water.

If you must drink alcohol, water it down or use more mixer. While I was quitting, I chose to drink Perrier or orange juice with a twist of lime and a swizzle stick. It looked like a highball and nobody made any challenging remarks.

The best drink of all is *water*.

• **Learn to love water.** To wake yourself up in the morning, have some water! I prefer it cold—a big glass of cold, clear water. Some people like to drink a cup of hot water with lemon first thing in the morning. That, too, really wakes you up—and gets your circulation and digestive system going—better than that first cigarette in the morning.

Water beats all the soft-drink promises to refresh—both

inside and out. Wash your hands and face with cool water, and then have a good glass of cold water. It's kinder to your poor overworked kidneys, too.

Water helps the kidneys flush out the hundreds of poisons that come with cigarette smoke, including, of course nicotine. The more water you drink, the faster your body will detoxify itself.

Altogether, water is a wonderful and inexpensive "treatment." If you don't have good-tasting water, buy spring water or one of those filter pitchers, for convenience. You deserve the best!

Water isn't a "cue" for a cigarette the way cola or coffee is—you can probably eliminate another couple of cigarettes just by substituting water for soda or coffee.

Water is a powerful *weight controller,* too. If you drink a glass of water before each meal, you won't eat as much. Your stomach will feel fuller sooner. It's also a super aid to regularity.

5. COMMAND YOURSELF TO GET SUFFICIENT REST. Reflect on the behavior of a child who is overtired. He becomes cranky, uncooperative, tense, unhappy. Then consider the difference in behavior when that child has had enough rest. Easy to get along with, high energy, happy. We adults are the same way. When we're tired, life gets tougher. When we're well-rested life becomes less pressured—it's easier to cope—which means you have less need to smoke.

So commit yourself to getting enough sleep for the next several weeks. Not too little or too much! That means getting to bed on time—staying up late is often a sign of childish rebellion—and getting up on time. Happily, when you stop smoking, you'll discover you wake up more easily and more refreshed.

It also means that you must do everything possible to insure sound sleep. I worked out a protocol for myself recently that works like a miracle for most people. In fact, many people who went through DietEnders field trials say the most exciting benefit was learning how to avoid sleeplessness. Here are several tricks to insure restful sleep:

• Never eat a heavy meal less than four hours before bed. "Heavy" means fatty, greasy foods, especially beef.

Because it's hard to digest, it's as if your stomach must keep the "factory" open for the late shift, when everybody is trying to get some sleep. Your heart is pumping hard to supply blood to your digestive tract, and all other body functions are working in high gear to get their share of the body's blood supply.

• Don't go to bed hungry. Have a light "supper" if necessary before bed. I like a Meal-In-A-Bag® with water, or some good complex carbohydrate and protein. For instance, a small portion of pasta and cottage cheese, or rice pudding or buckwheat groats (kasha) and milk. Obviously, *if you're concerned about weight gain* use low-fat cottage cheese, skim milk, little or no butter. These little suppers stick to our ribs because they digest slowly, so you don't have a drop in blood sugar during the night.

If you're not hungry before bed, have a glass of milk. It soothes your nerves and has lasting ability—to see you through the night.

If milk makes you "gassy," look for Lactaid milk, or buy "Lactaid" at the drug store.

• NEVER have sugar or sugary foods (simple carbohydrates) a couple of hours before bed. That means ice cream, candy, pies, cakes and cookies. It can wreck sleep in one of several ways: you might have trouble falling asleep, you might fall asleep for a couple of hours and then wake up and toss and turn, or you might have nightmares or weird dreams.

I had all these problems from time to time but now that I identified the cause I sleep like a baby. One common sign, caused by improper food intake, was that I would get itchy. My skin felt creepy. Even my face would get itchy! Observe yourself. If you have difficulty sleeping, reflect on what and when you ate. Then, if you hate bad sleep the way I do, you'll do everything you can to avoid it. (And when you're well rested you'll have an easier time coping and not smoking!)

• About a half hour before bed, take some fructose. (Then brush your teeth before going to sleep!) This insures that you have a steady flow of glucose in your blood stream all night long—even if you've excited your insulin with sugary foods, or if you have much on your mind and burn up glucose as you sleep. Once you work out your own needs, you can use the fructose only on an "as-needed basis." I wouldn't be without it now, although I don't use it often.

• Relax before bed. Instead of the news, which is purposely upsetting, watch some pleasant, amusing show, or turn on some soft music, or write in your journal. Remind yourself of your specialness. Review your workbook. Focus on good things you hope to achieve in the future . . . especially being free of cigarettes! Program your dreams in advance! (Try it. You'll be surprised at how often it works!) Say to yourself, "Tonight I want to dream a happy dream—of traveling somewhere exotic—or having fun with good friends—or being in love with a wonderful person . . ."

• Forgo napping during the day for a couple of days. Naps can set off a reactive chain of events which sometimes interferes with nighttime sleep. Although you may find yourself feeling drowsy for a few days after you quit smoking, you'll quickly be pleasantly surprised. You will very likely need less sleep when your body isn't fighting a poison. If you are drowsy during the day, take a catnap, or an Enerjet.

6. LEARN TO RELAX QUICKLY AND DEEPLY. We have a Relaxation Ritual in the SmokEnder and DietEnders programs in which we teach by demonstration and practice, but you can create a combination of the necessary elements for yourself in a routine that suits your own personal taste. Here are the elements:

• Take a slow, deep breath. Inhale through your nose and continue to inhale until you feel you have filled your diaphragm (the soft place below your ribs but above your navel). Think of it as a balloon. Try to bypass your lungs. You can't, of course, but it helps to visualize it that way. When you think you have taken in as much air as you can, take in some more. If you're doing it right, you'll feel a band of tightness around your back. As a smoker, you might cough when you do this, but very soon after you quit it will be smooth and easy.

• Exhale slowly through your mouth.

• As you inhale tighten each muscle, one by one. Hold it tight for three seconds, then exhale and relax. First your hands, then your arms, legs, feet, and so on.

• When all muscles are relaxed, put a dream picture in your mind—something soothing. Visualize yourself participating in that picture. Picture, for instance, a sailboat, with full sails gliding along on a calm sea. Concentrate on that image and nothing else. Stare at it in your mind's eye. Don't waver.

• This is a good time for you to add a sales pitch to yourself: Start with, "I really want to quit smoking. I CAN AND I WILL QUIT!" I know you don't fully believe that yet, but say it. It will soon be true!

• Visualize yourself as a nonsmoker. See yourself fresh and clean, glowing with radiant good health. (You'll be amazed at how quickly your body will restore itself.)

• Take another very deep breath. And another.

You will feel relaxed and refreshed—and will have eliminated the need for a few more cigarettes.

This really works. If you wonder about it, consider the effectiveness of advertising. How many products are you buying and using now that you didn't know existed before you saw them advertised? Why are you using them? Do you really need them? You were "programmed" to want them. You were convinced they were essential to your well-being or image—whatever. That's how advertising works.

Now "program" yourself to want to quit smoking. I assure you you can, if you care enough about yourself to take the time and make the simple effort necessary to know yourself, accept yourself and grow up that last little bit.

In addition to the Relaxation Ritual, you may want to use meditation as a means of relaxing. I recommend *The Relaxation Response,* by Herbert Benson, M.D. (Avon). Dr. Benson has demonstrated remarkable results with his techniques, including substantial reductions in blood pressure.

For wonderful relaxation, visualization, meditation books and cassettes, I recommend anything by Louise Hay or Shakti Gawain.

7. DON'T TAKE YOURSELF SO SERIOUSLY. Dust off your sense of humor. Every single thing you have responsibility for can't be earth-shaking. Let go of a few tasks and see what happens. You'll be surprised. You aren't all that important. . . .

8. SET REALISTIC PRIORITIES. By this time in your life you must realize that it's impossible to do everything that presents itself as an opportunity or responsibility. Successful time managers are ones who have learned to do the "Urgent and Important" tasks first—and to let the "Urgent but Unimportant" tasks pass.

When you have learned to hang loose and choose to be busy on *your* terms, you will have eliminated the need for a couple of cigarettes a day. Good for you!

9. GET YOUR CIRCULATION GOING. One of the best stress management techniques is physical movement. It acts as an escape valve—letting off steam—by rechanneling the hormonal changes caused by stress into a healthy outlet. It improves your physical stamina, which lets you handle stress more effectively. And it makes you feel good about yourself emotionally, because you know that you're really doing something good for yourself. For many it brings on a nice "high" when the brain chemicals flow. And without good circulation you can't have a healthy body. It's the circulating blood that freshens all your organs, nourishes, cleans, oxygenates and generally tidies up—carrying off dead materials and poisons like a good housekeeper.

Too often we're so sedentary that our circulation slows down, I suspect, to the speed of cold molasses. With a little encouragement, your circulation can pick up its pace and give you bonus benefits you may not have thought possible.

For instance, in addition to carrying off nicotine faster, improved circulation will put color in your cheeks (that's why a lot of smokers have a pasty pallor—smoking restricts the circulation to the surface of your skin); your bowel functions will become more regular; you'll start feeling better. And, as I said earlier, it will be easier to cope with stress.

How do you get your circulation going? There are hundreds of ways. Something to suit everyone, even those who hate to exercise. The secret is to find something you enjoy doing and make it a daily routine.

Don't start too ambitiously. Start at first with just five minutes a day . . . and build up gradually. And then, as Williams James, the father of modern psychology, said about habit formation, "never suffer an exception" to your practice of a new habit until it is ingrained.

Let me remind you that you're capable of making something a part of your life through habit: brushing your teeth is a learned behavior. You resisted at first, but your mother persevered, and now, very likely, you feel uncomfortable when you skip your toothbrushing routine.

To get started, I suggest you use the Karma Stretches at the back of the book. They are wonderful "warm-ups" designed for DietEnders by Karma Keintzler, exercise physiologist at Canyon Ranch Spa in Tucson, Arizona, and Lenox, Massachusetts. (A wonderful place. I recommend it. Consider it as a special reward for quitting smoking.) My daughter Lilla, an artist, translated the stretches graphically to make them easier to follow.

Do "Awake" for a few days and run in place for a total of just three minutes; then add "Aware" and make the total five or six minutes. There are five stretches in the set. You can improvise any good stretches, sit-ups and crunches to increase the time as you get into it.

Consider a "rebounder" (little trampoline) if you have bone or joint problems, or a stationary bicycle, weights, rowers, springs, etc. There are many good things available now, like treadmills and stairclimbers. Just be sure to try the equipment before you buy it to be sure it's right for you.

I keep my rebounder under the bed and pull it out while I watch TV now and then. I also bought a ten-speed bike with my cigarette money and on nice days, I ride outside.

There are some fine books to help you get started, too. I really recommend *Fit or Fat* by Covert Bailey (Houghton-Mifflin 1984). It's a very simple little book—and immensely motivating.

I also recommend yoga, aerobics, swimming, skiing (cross country and downhill) and, if you have a video recorder, Jane Fonda's or Joannie Greggin's workouts. They also come in audiocassette form, too, which is much less expensive and works well.

Another suggestion: check your TV listing to find a good yoga or aerobic program, and arrange your schedule accordingly, if possible—at least to get started.

There is one thing you can do that doesn't cost anything, doesn't hurt, gives sensational results and can be done anywhere: WALKING. If you aren't inclined to do any of the other suggestions, promise yourself you'll take a brisk walk every morning—or every lunchtime—or after work— whatever fits your schedule. The payoff is wonderful as a weight control and to lift depression. I bought myself a lightweight "Walkman"-type cassette player and listen to fast march music when I walk. It really gets me moving—and time goes so fast!

Start by walking about five minutes. Increase the time as you feel better about it. Try for thirty minutes a day. You'll soon enjoy it so much, you'll miss it if you don't walk.

Let me remind you that you should check with your doctor before starting any exercise program—especially if you are out of shape, over fifty, have any heart, muscle or joint problem.

Go for it. It's the best thing you can do for yourself short of quitting smoking.

10. PAMPER YOURSELF! Do nice things for yourself. Get into the habit of rewarding yourself with special treats. Take time off to read; take a walk, a bubble bath; visit or call a friend; spend some time on a favorite hobby; shop for something you'd like (within your budget; soon, after you stop smoking, you'll have thousands of dollars to spend on frivolous treats instead of on cigarettes.) The SmokEnder "Cost of Smoking" chart at the back of the book shows how much you'll "earn" by not smoking.

11. ADD SOME SPONTANEITY AND EXCITEMENT TO YOUR LIFE. Bob Conklin, in his book *Dynamics of Success* (Prentice-Hall), says that "Without 'expectation' you are mentally dead." He goes on to show how people who have no expectations accomplish very little and are dull. "Life is dull to people who are dull" is a common expression. And boredom is a big cause of smoking.

There are ways to alleviate loneliness and boredom. Making yourself important to other people is an obvious one. Find those who need your talents, experience, caring, time or money, if you have any extra, and help. You'll need good judgment to prevent yourself from becoming a busybody, an intruder or a dictatorial rich uncle. Take an interest in other people, sports, hobbies, etc.

12. DEAL WITH YOUR GUILT. Even when you're very busy, very much occupied with your work, with your family, friends, community, something can still seem to be missing. Consider for a moment the possibility that your smoking has placed a "smoke screen" between you and the joy and beauty of life. For some of us, the very fact that we know smoking is a form of self-destruction causes us to put life down. Guilt plays a strong hand. "Life can't be so great," we almost say, "or I'd cherish it and not risk it by smoking." Many smokers develop a blind spot to looking ahead over the years.

Now, this gets rather complicated, as I have learned from my own experience and from hundreds of smokers who have talked with me. Because we feel guilty about our smoking and "self-destruction," we lose some respect for ourselves each time we light up. I recall the case of a Supreme Court justice who went through the SmokEnder program some time ago. He was a very distinguished man; very much in control of his life, as you might imagine—except for his smoking. He said to me, "Jackie, you know I have attained a modicum of achievement in my field and I am respected for my accomplishment. People look up to me. But *I* don't!" He thought little of himself because he couldn't control his own smoking; he considered himself a fraud. After he quit smoking, he regained his self-respect and experienced a tremendous sense of liberation.

Guilt frequently spirals down to another human response that isn't too pretty. People often resort to martyr tactics in order to obtain reassurance that they are okay. They'll put themselves out for anyone, anytime. What they're really saying is, "I'm not so bad, am I? Look what I'm doing for you. Surely that proves that I have a lot of good in me." There are an infinite number of variations to this script. And people let you throw yourself under their feet as a doormat. They don't respect you for it—but you put yourself in the position of being available to be used. Why are you the one who drives the car pool so that everyone else can go to the big game? Why are you the last one in the office each night from your department? Why are you the one who scrapes the mud, carries the whole load, brings up the rear, stays outside to wait for the delivery while everyone else is inside having a good time? Why? Because you want to be a martyr and hope that someone will say, "What a dear person you are—so *good!*"

And because nobody says that, and nobody treats you with the respect you crave, you begin to feel sorry for yourself. Poor me! We're back to that again. So you light up to soothe your poor ego.

Let's do something about that!

A New Assurance

Let's yank the "smoke screen" away from your eyes. Reassure yourself that life is terrific, worth living. Take stock of what you're looking forward to. Make a list right now, and keep adding to it. Permit yourself a ray of hope that you will stop smoking soon and that when you do, the impetus of pride and confidence in your accomplishment will propel you to better things.

To get your engine warmed up, to help you overcome the inertia of breaking through the smoke screen that made life often seem dull and lifeless, here's a good lead.

Create expectations and surprises. That's a form of reward, too, but it takes a little help to get your creativity going to make it happen.

Bob Conklin asks us to use Mind Motivators to stir creativity. These Mind Motivators are simple questions, similar to those children ask. He asks us to open our eyes with expectation and wonder. Asking "why" and "what" begins a chain reaction of "I wish," and then "I will."

In the SmokEnder program we suggest to our smoker members that they plan new and interesting things they've never done before or haven't had time to do in a long time.

"What would I really like to do next time I have a half hour or a day free? What did I used to like to do that I haven't done in months? Years? Where can I go that will be refreshingly different?"

Keep a list of good ideas in your notebook so that you will remember them when you have some time. I still do that and am surprised at the number of fine ideas I've collected during the years.

Children have to see and touch and experience. Curiosity and the expectation of excitement are as much a part of childhood as growing. Somewhere through the years we buried all that. Why? To be sophisticated? Or because we're too busy?

Dig it out again! Fill your life with expectations and childlike adventures. When you stop smoking, you will have lovely habits with which to reward yourself. *The nicer you are to yourself the less you need to reward yourself with a cigarette.*

Now let's get back to the business of being a martyr.

The smoker who quits smoking successfully by following the SmokEnder concept of regaining self-respect and understanding the ego's involvement in smoking is certain to improve his self-esteem.

An early and visible sign of this is a self-assertiveness or independence on the part of the ex-smoker. The following observation was written by a 1969 SmokEnder graduate, Lois Rafalko, who later became a sensitive Moderator (teacher in the program) and successfully aided hundreds of smokers who attended her seminars in Pennsylvania. Her observations are based upon her own experience as a smoker—as a Moderator—and as a person exposed to vast amounts of smoking behavior.

"He [the ex-smoker] becomes unwilling to be imposed upon, intolerant of being taken for granted and will not, in any sense, be a martyr. This new assertiveness (usually noticed first by his immediate family) often represents an abrupt change in his behavior and may be misinterpreted by others (especially smokers) as irritability—due to kicking the habit.

"The SmokEnder may begin speaking out in situations where he previously remained quiet, though he may have seethed inside. For example, he may stand up to a wife (or husband or child) who has usually gotten her way . . . he may begin to complain about poor service or shoddy merchandise for which he is paying . . . he may even create a small scene in a supermarket over a man with a loaded grocery cart who is holding up an 'express' checkout line. He is asserting his own rights more firmly than before—because he has a new or stronger self-esteem.

"When this new attitude first rubs against people who are accustomed to the old behavior—it causes friction and other people tend to react by thinking, 'What's wrong with Joe?'

"One normally very shy and quiet SmokEnder, buoyed by her new victory over her smoking habit, found the courage to tell off a bully in the presence of a number of other people at a club meeting. When she got home from the meeting, she received several phone calls from friends, asking, 'What's wrong with you?' or 'Are you all right?'

"Members frequently hear remarks such as 'you're really irritable since you quit smoking' or 'why don't you have a cigarette to calm your nerves?'

"The danger here lies in the fact that if this situation is repeated often enough, the SmokEnder, himself, may begin to believe he is 'irritable' because he is not smoking. Sometimes members return to meetings after they stop smoking and say, 'I've been very irritable this week . . . my husband (or wife or child) tells me I've been very touchy (or edgy or snappish) since I quit smoking.'

"Smokers should be aware of this possibility; a smoker should understand the difference between his real motivation—self-respect—a positive trait, and nervous irritation, a negative one (which is common to those smokers who quit without proper preparation).

"If a smoker knows what is happening to him and why, no matter how often his mood is misinterpreted he will be able to see his behavior as a positive response and be reinforced by it."

So, surely, there's another big step in your self-knowledge. You must allow yourself to assert yourself—instead of smoking; and you must anticipate the jibes of friends and relatives in response to your newfound self-respect.

We discuss assertiveness and aggressiveness frequently in the program and clarify the difference between the two. So often people have picked up the habit of defensiveness and aggressiveness and wonder why life seems so tough. These are the people who have come to believe they must be direct and honest in their dealings with others—to a fault. Tact and diplomacy are out of their frame of reference. "I'll tell somebody they stink, if they do," I've heard a woman say. "Why would you tell them that?" I asked. "Well," she said, "because I believe in saying exactly what I think so people know where they stand with me."

This same woman, a prototype of many other men and

women I've dealt with in the SmokEnder program, later indicated that one of her problems is that she feels people are often against her. She was unable to develop the number of both casual and close friends she would have liked, and she couldn't understand why. Also, typical of the pattern, she bristled when anyone criticized her, first denying the criticism and then assaulting the critic.

The final stage of the pattern is repentance. She regretted immediately saying the things she had said and the tone of voice she had used, and very often she tried to repair the damage by being supersweet. I would say she was a passionate smoker—so many situations caused her to light up involuntarily. As I recall, this particular person smoked about two and a half packs a day for thirty years.

The happy ending is that she stopped smoking very comfortably—after she understood how immature her behavior was—and she stopped being defensive and became assertive rather than aggressive.

Courses in assertiveness training are still popular in many cities, and there are many books worth reading on the subject.

Before you can quit smoking comfortably, you will want to reduce a number of unnecessary stressful situations caused by difficulties with interpersonal relationships.

Reward/Guilt/Martyrdom

It is important that we understand how the reward concept relates to the "need" to smoke, in order to expose self-pity, martyrdom and guilt, so I will repeat some earlier concepts.

The "need" to smoke grows out of an addiction to nicotine and becomes a compulsion. The addictive need is then augmented by a second "need": to react repeatedly as a result of conditioned responses that have developed concurrently. The third need that emerges is the need for an escape valve, for self-expression, for recognition and ultimately for reward. It is this third area which requires further examination.

Eric Berne, M.D., in his book *Games People Play*, presents one explanation for this "recognition-reward" need. He suggests that infantile stimulus-hunger emerges into a pattern of behavior that he calls "recognition-hunger." This can be satisfied by "stroking"—a term generally used to mean intimate physical contact (such as the stroking or patting of a baby). Dr. Berne extends this term to mean any act that implies recognition of another's presence. A "stroke" may be thought of as the fundamental unit of social action. (Smokers may well be using each cigarette as a "stroke," a counterfeit means of satisfying the need induced by recognition-hunger—or, in other words, of satisfying one's ego.)

We all need some form of stroking—praise, a pat on the back, appreciation: a reward to confirm how good we are, to confirm that we exist. This recognition for which we hunger comes all too rarely. Our boss, our mate, our children and our colleagues usually complain to us much more than they thank us or express appreciation. As a result, we may have narcissistically conferred the property of "reward" upon our cigarette (as the ads tell us)—the pat on the back that says, "You've done a really good job." It isn't much, but a smoker is willing to settle for it.

"Smoking" does not recognize your goodness. In fact, it really makes most smokers feel guilty because they know it is self-destructive. When we have this guilt, we feel we deserve punishment; in an attempt to assuage the guilt and to gain the approval that will shore up our self-respect, the smoker may become a willing martyr.

As smokers, we must learn to reward ourselves in a less self-defeating way, but we cannot achieve this until we feel good about ourselves. Motivations and needs are always changing. The smokers' needs change as they go through the quitting process. We must be taught to handle these changing needs and encouraged to quit smoking for ourselves because we like ourselves. Therefore, in the Smok-Ender program, the Moderator leads the smoker through the following paces:

1. You're no longer a child, so stop seeking external recognition.
2. You will think better of yourself and throw off guilt when you quit smoking.
3. As self-image improves, self-pity is eliminated and self-respect returns.

4. Self-satisfaction becomes the ultimate reward, since you are doing something for yourself because you like yourself.

The smoker learns he doesn't need external recognition anymore. When he has done a good job, he can feel proud. That is *internal* recognition. It is having grown up. And when he needs confirmation of his existence, his polished, shiny, clean new ego will give him that reassurance. It is then that he will really be his own person. He can truly be free and not need to smoke!

Don't Smoke—Stroke! There's nothing like a strong dose of honest self-mastery to enhance one's image of oneself. This spirals upward into a form of self-respect which can't be bought. And the upward success spiral "infects" other areas of your life so that you welcome new challenges. You become a winner.

8

What the Cigarette Companies Knew . . . And When They Knew It

(Ads, Bans and Taxes)

As I write this update, 1994, the multibillion-dollar world of tobacco is in a shambles. At last. (Except in poor-developing countries, where the tobacco industry is vigorously marketing their particular form of death and disease—an American shame.)

In the United States, smoking has become socially unacceptable; new state and federal taxes are being imposed daily, the Food and Drug Administration will regulate tobacco advertising and marketing, if not nicotine content; forty-four states and the District of Columbia now restrict smoking in public places; major league ball parks, many fast foot chains, and one-third of the nation's malls are going smokeless; OSHA (Occupational Safety and Health Administration) is preparing to ban smoking in virtually *all* buildings in the country, except private homes; there is talk in Congress about finally eliminating tobacco price support and subsidies; a $5 billion class action suit is being filed against the tobacco companies on behalf of everyone who has ever been addicted; Mississippi and Florida are suing the industry for the Medicaid cost due to smoking; and the Surgeon General's report concluded that nicotine is as addictive as heroin and cocaine.

Still, the cigarette industry denies there's a relationship between smoking and illness, *and* that nicotine is addictive. At a congressional hearing this spring, seven chief executives of tobacco companies testified, under oath, one after another, "I believe nicotine is not addictive." It was almost laughable—except it concerns you and me, and our children, and all those who have died and who will yet die *prematurely* from smoking-related diseases.

In addition, they are accused of manipulating nicotine levels in cigarettes to keep us truly hooked, and it has been proven that they knew in the mid-fifties that nicotine is addictive, but suppressed research showing smoking's addictive effects. They claim they use nicotine to improve taste. Although they have decreased the tar and changed flavoring additives over the years, they have never lowered the average nicotine level!

Taste, indeed. (In a later chapter you will go on a Taste Hunt. The results are informative.)

That they have been able to freely market a highly addictive drug, a product that when used as intended will cause disease and premature death, is a national disgrace.

When I finally took a willing look at the problem, in 1968, about 67% of Americans smoked. We were in the majority. Cigarettes were marketed in the most outrageous uncontrolled way: free cigarettes were handed out in the streets, mailed to "occupant" in millions of homes (and kids often got their first smokes that way!), were freely given to service men (most started to smoke in the service), and later were sold for pennies at ship's stores and commissaries; TV advertising was at an all-time high—the biggest advertiser on the air. Tobacco was off limits to the FDA (and still is, but hopefully not for long). But everyone looked the other way when anyone spoke of taking action to limit the epidemic of smoking-related disease.

The tobacco lobby is the richest in Washington, and until

recently, the most powerful. It still has great power, but voters now know the enormous burden smoking places on the cost of health care—a big issue in the U.S. They also know, now, that secondhand smoke is dangerous to non-smokers.

The word has reached Congress: Smoking is BAD for the economy. It's bad for non-smoker's health. (The argument that tobacco farmers would suffer economically if smoking were banned is fallacious: First, they can grow other crops on their land or learn other skills and trades. Second, who cried for the harness makers when automobiles came on the scene? Those who were enterprising made leather car seats; those who hid from reality were lost. Third, there is now foreign competition—from China, Zimbabwe, Brazil, and Argentina—and they're selling at one-half to two-thirds of American prices. (*N.Y. Times* 8/28/94) Of course, the tobacco industry is deserting the American tobacco farmers.

The argument that taxes would be lost if people stopped smoking is also incorrect: the excess health care costs—billions per year for Medicaid and Medicare—far exceed any tax revenue received to this writing.

Among the proposals to fund universal health care is a big federal tax on cigarettes. Here's a staggering fact: There are fifty million smokers in the U.S. The average smoked is one and a half packs a day. If they pay an additional tax of a dollar per pack per day, that's $75 million A DAY! That's a lot of health care.

Quite a paradox: Many smokers will quit because of sticker shock, so the total tax collected will be less than projected. BUT, since the body restores itself quickly after cessation, medical care, medication and hospitalization due to smoking will be sharply reduced, so the cost of health care will go down. Much better for all concerned. Except the cigarette manufacturers.

Not to worry about them. They have been marketing aggressively to developing countries like Indonesia and China, where about 70% of the men smoke. For years they have been sending cigarettes to poor nations under the Food for Peace program! Outrageous. (Yet the FDA was unable to consider cigarettes as a food or a drug. See below.)

It was political suicide for a congressman, senator, cabinet officer or any elected official to speak out against tobacco. (It's still unhealthy, politically, for many legislators from tobacco-growing states.)

Perhaps worst of all, somehow the tobacco industry had held hostage scientists, health agencies, government health departments, medical and dental societies as far as addiction was concerned. For example, in 1906, cigarette manufacturers made a deal with Congress to exclude tobacco from control by the FDA.

This is what a heroic Dr. David Kessler, M.D., LLD, the FDA commissioner, is trying to undo. He has proof that nicotine is addictive and therefore a drug, which falls under his jurisdiction. The problem is, Dr. Kessler doesn't want to have it listed under the FDA because that would force him to ban cigarettes in the U.S.—and that would leave fifty million smokers screaming for relief, and attacking their legislators. Worse, it would create a major black market and the attendant underworld crime.

He wants Congress to pass a law giving the FDA control over advertising, marketing and content. Ultimately, they suggest, a cigarette with no nicotine could be made. Alas, without the kick of nicotine, most smokers would not buy those brands. They'd find "real" cigarettes.

A non-nicotine cigarette would at least prevent children from getting hooked when they make their first few tries at smoking. Now, with high-nicotine brands—a favorite among kids—a few cigarettes for a short time and they're hooked!

Internationally

France. Forty percent are smokers. Laws restricting smoking in most public places, and a prohibition on all tobacco advertising.

Britain banned advertising on TV in 1965; in 1971 was one of the first to require health warnings on packs.

Germany. Non-smoking train cars and smoke-free areas in restaurants.

Italy. Smoke-free theaters and public transportation, with new laws in the works for hospitals and schools.

Singapore. Tough laws against smoking. No smoking in public places, no cigarette vending machines and no sponsorship of public events. Singapore hopes to become the world's first smoke-free city.

China. Seventy percent of the men are smokers. Bans advertising and restricts smoking in public places, even though it is the world's largest producer and consumer of tobacco.

Hong Kong. Imposed a 300% tax on cigarettes in 1983, and another 100% in 1993.

Japan. Sixty-percent of adult males smoke. Non-smoking areas in workplaces. (*Time* 11/23/92)

We don't yet know how much the tobacco industry spends to attract smokers abroad, but the staggering fact is they spent over five *billion* in 1992 on advertising and promotion in the United States. Keep in mind, the focus of their advertising often seems to be adolescents and minors—they need new smokers to replace those thousands who die or quit each year, and kids are their target.

The Joe Camel campaign is particularly onerous: in 1988, just before R. J. Reynolds introduced the cartoon character, Joe Camel, the Camel brand had only 0.5% share of the "illegal" market—children under eighteen years old. That represented about $6 million in sales. In 1991, only four years after the introduction of Joe Camel, market share of sales to kids increased to 32.8% and sales of Camels was $476 million.* Yet the tobacco industry insists they don't advertise to attract children, just to persuade adults—like you?—to change brands. Remarkably, the Federal Trade Commission agreed, finding in 1994 that they had not seen proof that the ads convinced children to smoke.

Now let's look at the cigarette ads from the tobacco industry's point of view. The cigarette companies have really done a superb job of marketing their product. Can you imagine persuading sixty to seventy million people to do something that costs money; that's kind of dirty; that makes them smell bad; that usually offends friends and relatives; that causes gagging and coughing, slows them down, is in general a pretty messy nuisance and might kill them?

I give the tobacco industry and its advertising agencies

---

*DiFranza, *Journal of American Medical Assn.*, Dec. 11, 1991.

credit for doing a tremendous job. I don't like what they do, because I've seen the wrong end of it for many years—early death, and the daily pain and anguish smokers experience from knowing their suffering has been self-inflicted.

But it's not my role to hassle the tobacco industry or act like "hatpin Annie"—we in SmokEnders are not vindictive and we're not interested in wasting effort and energy on vendettas. The objective is to help people break free from the smoking habit if they have decided they'd like to quit. This book is intended to motivate you to want to quit—and then to guide you to success. But it's important to have a good, clear view of the propaganda and not continue to let the ads reach you even subliminally.

I can hear you say, "Oh, the ads don't get me. I'm not moved by them; I don't even see them, really. I'm too sharp for that!" Sure you are, except that I don't believe it because I said it myself, too, and I was in the advertising business as a young woman and prided myself on being astute about advertising messages. And yet the ads influenced me, though I didn't know to what length and depth until I stopped smoking.

So let's talk about the approach the tobacco industry took to lead us into its domain. Let's turn the tables by using the ads to get disengaged from the habit.

Early on their approach was "Reward yourself. Treat yourself to something special." "For a treat instead of a treatment" was no accident. Advertising copywriters understand human nature—and human needs. Our need for recognition is fully discussed in Chapter 7.

The next exercise, something you'll enjoy, is rather like exorcising a devil. If that sounds dramatic, forgive me, but I know how strongly the cigarette ads are imprinted upon your mind, whether or not you know it yet. Let me try to make my point.

Suppose smoking were required by a government decree, like taxes or payroll reports. Can you imagine the uproar? There would be a rebellion. Not just because it violated our rights and forced us to do something against our will, but because it is such a dangerous and disgusting activity. And no amount of advertising would persuade us that it could be good for us, that it would improve the economy, that we might learn to like it.

So what has given us all the idea that smoking is a pleasure, that it creates a desirable image? *We were programmed.* It hasn't always been so. Cigarettes were a minor commodity until World War I, when they were issued to soldiers as a gesture of kindness. But they didn't gain public acceptance on a large scale until years later, when some brilliant advertising minds realized they had to aim at the "beautiful" people. Instead of directing their advertising efforts toward the tobacco-chewing crowd from which their customers were largely drawn, they consciously and vigorously portrayed smoking as "smart" and sophisticated, something done by the much-admired "upper class." In terms of changing public opinion, the new advertising direction was a huge success. The rest is history. The ads struck the nerve, were right on target. People forced themselves to smoke since it was so "in." The ads kept telling our parents that they couldn't make it unless they smoked. And they smoked in great numbers.

I'm going to tell you how to translate the ads so that they work *for* you instead of against you. The early ads took a slick, sophisticated approach; the current ones show machismo and "cool" and "taste"—both meanings.

Here's how to read the ads. It's something we teach in the SmokEnders program, which is fun and effective. You'll soon get the hang of it and never again be subject to their subtle manipulation. What we do is parody the ads. If you change one thing, it will change the whole meaning. A favorite of mine is the ad that showed a rather angry-looking young man with his shirt open to his navel, a neck chain and the proper accessories of his generation that represent "cool." The copy announces, "I like the box!" This can be read in several ways—take your choice. Either the boy prefers to smoke the box or he is referring to an off-color meaning of "box." In either case, he's not selling cigarettes. What about the fellow who's been scuba-diving with heavy equipment? He's sitting on the edge of a boat and reaching for a cigarette. This should read "I can't dive 'cause I smoke; just don't have the wind." Or how about the young lady who says, "If it weren't for _____, I wouldn't smoke"? Except when she runs out of that brand, she'll smoke "Others" brand—anything else she can get her hands on. She's hooked!

And Mr. Cowboy. Why that should sell cigarettes is hard to understand unless you catch what underlies it: ego, machismo, toughness, "cool," all things kids desire. Change the copy to read "Come to Cancer Country." This is what a British TV outfit did. It asked permission to film the famous cowboys for a documentary on effective advertising. It interviewed cowboys who had been stricken with lung cancer, emphysema and other smoking-induced diseases. The program was a knockout, though very embarrassing to the company.

Right now there are a great number of low-tar cigarettes on the market. Their copy implies that they are "safer." But safer than what? Read their ads and laugh. Each one promises less tar than the next, though *Reader's Digest* proclaims that low-tar brands produce considerably more poisonous gas than regular brands. And one new ad asserts that brand _____ has less poisonous gas than other brands. Read these ads as a confession from the tobacco industry. "These are *less* damaging than other brands . . ." How funny that they have been so caught up in the race for sales—with their internal bickering—that they're hanging their dirty laundry out in public.

I'm reminded of the old ads—when cigarettes were first found to have a link with cancer. The ads tumbled off the presses declaring that each brand was "less irritating" or "cooler on the throat" or contained a more effective filter which sifted out a lot of the dangerous elements.

Let's face it. There is nothing good one can really say about cigarettes in print. When you take time out to think about the words the copywriters use and not the pictures, you soon realize that they can't think of anything to say (without breaking the law).

Have you seen the ad about the man who has just won $25,000, has poured a bucket of champagne over his head and is certainly not going to follow all that with a "boring" cigarette? You have to picture him lighting up, fireworks coming out of his cigarette, as a brass band plays "The Stars and Stripes Forever." Well, you have to admit, that would be exciting.

Or you see a picture of an intense young man with beautiful hair and a beard, looking at you straight on and

saying, "If I'm going to smoke, I'm going to do it right."
Your imagination can really take off on that one. "First, I
must extract the cigarette from the pack without bending it;
then I must be sure not to put the tobacco end in my mouth
and light the filter tip; and I certainly want to be careful not
to singe my beard. Today I'm going to do it right."

Do smokers always dress in color-coordinated outfits of
the latest style, and wrinkleless? Are smokers perfectly
groomed, their nails gorgeously manicured? Most ads show
us smokers who are youthful, slender, with a glow of good
health and well-being: laughing, horsing around in the water
(how do they keep their cigarettes dry?), having loads of
fun. How many of us really look like that?

You should pay attention to what is really being said.
Many of the words are what is known in the trade as "weasel
words": words that are evasions or retreats; words that
either mean nothing or imply something that isn't true. One
of the big weasel words is "helps," which in fact means aids
or assists. What the ad is saying, as it uses that word, is that
the product doesn't actually do what it claims to do, it only
partially does it. "The filter *helps* trap gas." The ad neglects
to tell you the names of the gases because they are lethal
poisons, and you probably won't want to smoke a poisonous
product. Poisons like carbon monoxide (you know, like
from out of the back of your car?) and hydrogen cyanide
are examples.

"Like" is another "weasel word" that confuses. *Like*
invokes comparison—something may seem to be one thing,
but in fact really isn't. "Draws like a gentle breeze." Have
you ever drawn in a gentle breeze?

And what about "taste," which is a purely subjective
daydream of the copywriters? Who can say that a cigarette
has the "taste" of "iced lightning" unless perhaps you've
tasted iced lightning. Then there are "smooth taste" and
"cool taste," the "taste of fresh menthol" (another ingredient that is causing suspicion these days)—how, one wonders, does that compare with *stale* menthol? There are the
taste of adventure, the taste of all outdoors, a "taste that is
very real" (is there a taste that is very phony?). And why all
these euphemisms? Does anyone ever say a cigarette tastes
like tobacco? No, because as I said before, cigarettes do

taste lousy most of the time, and if the ads admitted that cigarettes tasted like tobacco, who would want to smoke them?

If one were to substitute the word "cigarettes" for the name of a specific brand that is heavily promoted, the copy would read, "If it weren't for cigarettes, I wouldn't smoke."

We often imagine how cigarette commercials might appear if they were still permitted on television. David Ballantine, a friend with a lively imagination, dreamed up this scenario: An ambulance is seen racing through the night—lightning, thunder, flashing red lights, sudden stop in front of a massive building. Attendants run around to the back of the ambulance. Doors are flung open. An unusually beautiful blond woman is lifted out on a stretcher. She is wearing expensive jewelry and is covered with a gold-lamé blanket. Camera pans to front of building. "Memorial Cancer Institute" is visible on the stone lintel above the door. Voice-over: "You've come a long way, baby." Realizing that there is nothing good to say about cigarettes can make ad watching a self-reinforcing activity.

It is most curious that cigarette manufacturers are now obliged by law to spend 2% of their advertising space and advertising dollars to warn you off their product! "Warning: The Surgeon General has determined that cigarette smoking is dangerous to your health" and five other explicit warnings (but none yet about addiction) must be prominently displayed on ads, billboards and packaging. Is there another consumer product that says "this product is dangerous to your health" that we would buy? Butter? A mattress? A child's toy? How about dog food? Would we ever buy a can of dog food that stated unequivocally on the label, "Warning, this food is bad for the health of your dog"?

It is also interesting that, at the last count, there were several hundred varieties of cigarettes on the American domestic market, and nearly all of them are manufactured by six major companies. It's fairly obvious that the company that makes the best ads—not the best cigarettes—wins.

At SmokEnders we point out that ads don't really influence which cigarette you smoke. How many times have you as a smoker actually changed your brand over the past twenty years? Once? Perhaps twice? Many ads imply that smoking a certain brand of cigarette will add tremendous sex appeal, because those are the ads that have the best-looking models, who exude sensuality and suggest that all you need to emulate them is to smoke their brand. How much sex appeal can you have if your hair and body smell of stale smoke, if you have nicotine-stained teeth and fingers, if your breath reeks? There is also evidence that smoking inhibits sexual performance. Our graduates have often alluded to the fact that stopping smoking had had an opposite effect. *Subliminal Seduction* by Wilson Bryan Key points out that cigarette ads are filled with sexual imagery and phallic symbols. The consumer is supposed to be defenseless against such enticements. Still, smoking a cigarette waxes pale in comparison with the real thing.

Cigarette advertising campaigns of the 1930s and forties seem primitive in the light of what we know today about smoking. It was a time when the medical profession was somewhat naive about the dangers of smoking and doctors were even known in some cases to *recommend* smoking to patients who were nervous, or who wanted to lose weight. Cigarette advertising went to great lengths to assume a medical seal of approval, figuratively speaking. One brand actually claimed statistically that "20,679 Physicians say" that the particular brand was "less irritating because 'It's toasted' " (the advertiser's quotes around 'It's toasted,' immediately lead to suspicion). Then the copy went on to say that this toasting was "Your Throat Protection against irritation and against cough," that "Toasting removes dangerous irritants that cause throat irritation and coughing." This was before filter tips, an innocent age. One could, in any event, thus naturally assume that if your doctor smoked a particular cigarette, then it really had to be good for you.

Approach cigarette ads with a fresh point of view. You'll probably find that they help you get ready to stay off cigarettes. When you read the ad that asks, "If smoking isn't a pleasure, why bother?" you may say, "You know, it *isn't* a pleasure; I guess I *won't* bother!" Another connection disconnected!

If you want to do it right, begin tearing out ads and leave them around until you have a good idea of how to change the meaning. If there are children around, they do marvels with this. I remember one time our son Peter, then about ten, found a typical ad of the lovely young lady sitting by a cool pool, looking fresh and pure, holding a cigarette in her hand, waiting expectantly for Mr. Wonderful, who was emerging from the background. Ah, what promise of joy and pleasure were implied! Peter destroyed the image with one move of his pencil. He blackened one of her front teeth.

When you have created a good parody, you might hang it on your refrigerator for the whole family to enjoy. It does a good job in helping youngsters learn to "read" the ads. Satire is a marvelous tool to prevent children from starting to smoke.

9

Changing Other Habits
(What About Alcohol, Cola, Coffee and Recreational Drugs?)

Invariably I'm asked, "Now that I've kicked the cigarette habit would there be any risk if I smoked something else"—a recreational drug? They're not asking my advice about drugs, but want to know if it will risk relapse to cigarettes.

Of course, it's sensible to avoid any possibility of resuming smoking once one has finally quit. So, ideally, we should sidestep alcohol, too, and coffee, Coke/Pepsi and almost any other substance that acts as a "trigger" for a cigarette. I've met hardly any smokers who haven't been tied to the combination of cigarette-and-coffee; cigarette-and-liquor; cigarette-and-Coke. We have records of smokers who have consumed up to thirty cups of coffee a day or about twenty bottles of Coke a day while they were smokers—and when they stopped smoking their caffeine intake dropped dramatically; and many near-alcoholics have reported they reduced their alcohol intake considerably, in some cases totally.

Stopping smoking, they also broke the conditioned-response "command" and found they didn't need to drink coffee, Coke or alcohol as much as before.

In addition, because they weren't drugged by nicotine and all the gases which slowed them down mentally and physically while they were smoking, they found they didn't need the lift or release which those cigarette "companions" seemed to offer. In fact, the sense of being turned on is remarkably strong when one stops smoking correctly, well prepared to walk coolly and graciously away from the habit, so we don't require other means to get turned on as much as when we smoked tobacco.

But life is not perfect, and sometimes we need a kick. So for those who want to smoke something else now and then after they've kicked the habit, we caution them to avoid it until they are well away from the cigarette habit—until they have come to enjoy not-smoking as a pleasure which they wouldn't want to give up. Once that attitude is achieved, it's reasonable to assume that one could smoke a joint, for instance, with sufficient disassociation from the cigarette condition that it wouldn't trigger off a desire for a regular cigarette. That's the real problem. It's also a matter of re-solve.

In order to have quit successfully, you will have convinced yourself that you really wanted to quit; that there was something in it for you personally and that you're worth it. This resolve becomes stronger and stronger as you success-fully pass by each condition that used to remind you of a cigarette. Your self-esteem increases and, with it, your re-solve.

It takes considerable practice to become an experienced ex-smoker just as it took practice to become an experienced smoker. During the practice stage of not-smoking—for a period of time after you've quit—your resolve is vulnerable. You might even occasionally forget the reason you wanted to quit. And then, there are times when your resolve is softened by chemical forces—alcohol, for instance.

Let's look at the effects of alcohol on your system when you are a smoker and when you are a non-smoker. Since your body maintains a level of nicotine (generally a stimu-lant) while you support the cigarette habit, the effect of alcohol (generally a depressant) is reduced. When you stop smoking, alcohol functions at full strength and packs a much stronger wallop. (This could be a nice additional reason for wanting to quit smoking: you will need less to achieve the same feeling. This observation has been reported to us by numerous SmokEnder graduates.)

Here's the peril: when you have a drink, or use a drug, it softens the resolve. You adopt an "I don't give a damn" attitude, and the chances of reaching for a cigarette are vastly increased. I'd be willing to bet that more people start smoking again because they were caught off guard by alcohol's new kick, or pot's ability to "take the edge off things," than for almost any other reason.

So the answer to "What about recreational drugs now that I've kicked the cigarette habit?" is, if you want to protect your precious new habit of not-smoking, steer clear for a while. And by all means go easy on the alcohol. You'll find you really don't need to drink so much or so often because you don't have a cigarette that needs a companion—a drink. And because you will have come to realize that you don't need to follow old patterns just from habit. Stopping smoking is a catalyst for getting out of other ruts.

In fact, one of the pleasantest results of quitting was reported by a Greenwich, Connecticut, advertising executive. He had completed the SmokEnder course about six months before. "Dear Mrs. Rogers," he wrote, "I can't begin to tell you how much your program has done for me. Not only have I quit smoking very comfortably, which I thought was totally impossible for a person in my position and industry, but I have rearranged some other very important conditions in my life."

He described some rather touching personal situations in his life, including a drinking ritual. Without ever questioning why, he had had a couple of drinks at lunch and three martinis before dinner. He had steadily increased his alcohol consumption over the years. Then, in his late forties, he had observed that life had taken a downturn; things weren't exciting lately. He had begun to ask himself that question many people ask as they lift up their heads and look around after about forty years of pressing on through school and marriage and a career: "Is this all there is?"

"I found my life was becoming a boring routine. Rat race all day—same problems, different people. At night, I'd generally get home for a late dinner, after a couple of relaxing drinks, and stumble into bed so I could get up to go through the same routine in the morning. I'd say to myself, 'What's it all about?' "

Then he described the change he had made in his life-style, after his SmokEnder Moderator had taught him to determine if his routine might be an impediment now.

"That silly little 'ham story' you use in the program to persuade us to look at our lifestyle and patterns objectively really did the trick for me," he wrote. "I recognized that I could change much about my routine if I chose to. So I did. I realized that I didn't need those drinks at lunch anymore. The reason I got into that routine in the first place was because as a young man at my first job in New York, having a cocktail at lunch was a sign of 'belonging' to the fast-moving, sophisticated advertising clique. Everyone did it. The ritual. A vodka gimlet or a vodka martini at lunch was big stuff. (The reason it had to be vodka was because it left no odor on my breath.) Ordering two drinks at lunch took some years of development and signified another level of achievement for us. It let the world know that we could hold our liquor—two cocktails would 'snogger' ordinary types. And it expressed our financial status to the world. We could afford to squander our salary; two cocktails were expensive for a file clerk but not for a rising young executive.

"Then after I married, Madeleine and I followed the script of the scene as we had read it and seen it portrayed in plays, movies and books. It was another note of sophistication to have cocktails ready when I came home from the office. At first it got in the way of doing the things I looked forward to doing when I got home—like mowing the lawn or finishing the antique chest we had bought on our honeymoon. Soon I learned to stop promising myself I'd get things done in the evenings. That's what Saturdays are for, they told me at the office.

"And soon Madeleine became busy with the children, so we added a second cocktail to the routine to give her a bit more time to get dinner ready. Eventually it became three before dinner for me, because I'd stop at the Biltmore for a drink with Harvey before we took our separate trains at Grand Central. Dinner was always late, so I had extra time.

"And my evenings were all the same, unless we had friends over. A couple of drinks, a late dinner, watch the news on TV and then to bed.

"I simply accomplished nothing between leaving the office and going to bed. And I always complained that I didn't have time to get anything done that was pressing me.

"Sure, I carried home a briefcase full of work, but unless there was a critical deadline, I rarely worked in the evening.

"So when Ruth Sussman, my Moderator, suggested we take a cold, hard look at our patterns and routines and see if we had created some 'self-imposed jails and ruts,' I thought about that old wooden chest I had started to refinish. And I thought about the wasteland of my evenings, and I understood what Ruth was aiming at.

"As a result of quitting smoking, I've also cut down on my alcohol intake and have added four hours a day to my existence, because I don't have three cocktails before dinner. Now, we have an earlier dinner and I'm raring to go instead of being heavy-headed and tired. I look forward to the evenings as a time to spend on things I enjoy.

"I wish someone had told me years ago that I didn't have to play out the scenario of the Hollywood/Broadway stereotype of a sophisticate. So your program did far more for me than simply help me kick the habit. It improved the quality of my life beyond belief, for which I extend my most sincere appreciation."

Here's the "ham story" which influenced our friend and many others to repattern their lives:

A newly married couple decided to invite their parents to dinner as their first try at having company. They planned and shopped very earnestly, and then the proud young husband watched his bride prepare the meal. They had decided on baked ham, and after she had completed preparing it for the roasting pan, she sliced a chunk off one end and put it in the roasting pan next to the ham.

"Why did you do that, honey?" he asked.

"Oh," she said, "I honestly don't know. That's the way my mother always did it."

Perplexed, he asked his mother-in-law at dinner that evening, "Why did you always cut the end off the ham?"

"You know, I really don't know, come to think of it. But my mother always did it, and I never thought too much about it," she said.

The young husband was curious, and the next time they called on Grandma he remembered to ask her why she had cut the end off the ham. He wondered if it was a religious custom or had something to do with flavor.

"Good Lord, no," she said. "I cut the end off the ham because my roasting pan wasn't big enough."

Alcohol: Here's a suggestion for decreasing the amount of alcohol you consume without feeling deprived. Water it down. Whatever it is you drink (except beer, of course), you can add more mixer or soda or ice. When the day comes that you quit smoking, you won't have *two* big things to deal with. Also, one of the bonuses of stopping smoking is that you'll get a bigger kick from the same amount of alcohol.

Coffee: This is an interesting side condition. Our consumption of coffee is related directly to the number of cigarettes we smoke. So when we quit we discover that we have considerably reduced our coffee drinking, we are less keyed up. Also, you will save a considerable amount of time. Following the well-described routine of your day (and that of *most* smokers), you know there's a lot of stopping for coffee. One of our first members, Marilyn Durham, who now lives in Oregon, described her attachment to coffee while she smoked. She drank thirty cups of coffee a day: she had a fifteen-cup coffeepot in which she brewed coffee twice each day. After she completed the seminar, not only had she quit smoking and cut down her coffee to about five cups a day, but she had a lot more time. "In fact," she said, "I feel like somebody took the pressure off my life. Everything is calmer and less frenzied. I seem to get my work done in half the time and still have time to loaf or do the things I enjoy without feeling like my work is backing up on me."

The problem of coffee nerves disappears, and with it go all the stalling and indecision represented by the coffee ritual. Here's how it works. (I call it the Sunday-morning planning session, because that's how it was with me.) Sunday morning: We look forward to a day of pleasure and doing all those good things we've waited for all week. Everybody has high hopes for the day. First, though, we have to have breakfast talk over coffee about what we're going to do. Each cigarette demands another cup of coffee, and each cup of coffee requires another cigarette. The discussion is prolonged "just until I finish my cigarette," or "just until I finish this cup of coffee." The two never quite get into sync.

The morning is wasted, the kids are cranky because they are anxious to do whatever they had hoped to do with the family and by the time we get our act together, most of the precious day is gone.

A lot of the Monday-morning blues is a hangover of a disappointing Sunday.

Many of us repeat the ritual in miniature each time we stop for a coffee break, or a Coke or a cup of tea. It seems to be worse for those at home than for those in an office. We did a random sampling of smokers to determine how much time they spent drinking coffee each day. They were asked to list the time they spent drinking coffee and working simultaneously, and the amount of time they spent drinking coffee as a means of taking a break or socializing. Not counting breakfast, lunch and dinner coffee, the response ranged from thirty minutes to two hours a day. Measuring this against the habits of nonsmokers, we discovered that the latter spent about 55% less of their time drinking coffee for a "break."

There's a whole area of habits to explore in an effort to understand yourself in order to get ready to quit smoking successfully. That's the whole question of other drugs which you may be introducing into your system each day, not really thinking about the problems they create. Coffee is one of them. Or a "non-drug," as Edward Brecher, in his book *Licit and Illicit Drugs* (Consumer Reports—Little, Brown), classifies caffeine. "Nonmedically, caffeine is the most widely used central nervous system stimulant, popular in the form of coffee, tea, cocoa, and 'cola' drinks. Heavy users of these beverages report tolerance, physical dependence and withdrawal symptoms, and craving."

But never mind trying to decide whether you must abstain

from all pleasures if you quit smoking. The answer is no. I sincerely believe you should be able to quit smoking and simply disengage your smoking habit from your other habits without too much disturbance. In fact, in whatever form you take your caffeine, you should *be very careful not to cut down too sharply too quickly,* or you'll suffer caffeine withdrawal.

In the meantime, here are a couple of thoughts to help you out.

Substitute bouillon for several of the breaks. Keep a few packages in your pocket or your desk. I prefer the powdered kind in the foil packet. Very small. Very tasty. And it dissolves in hot water. When you feel like a good, hot pickup, try bouillon. It has helped a large number of smokers in the program. It contains protein, which gives you a boost, and it's soothing, rather than stimulating. Many of the brands contain sodium, so if you've on a limited diet, discuss it with your doctor, or find one of the low-sodium brands.

The other suggestion is to be aware that coffee is a mild diuretic. If you cut down sharply, you might find yourself feeling bloated. Sometimes you retain fluid until the body makes the necessary adjustments to handle the fluid without benefit of caffeine. If you find you're feeling "swollen"— perhaps your rings feel tight, or your shoes—the cause might be your reduction in coffee. If that's the case, there's nothing to worry about because it will pass. You can help it along by eating such things as mushrooms, spinach or asparagus, which are natural diuretics. Or ask your doctor for a suggestion.

Cut down your caffeine intake slowly. Use milk, water or bouillon as an occasional substitute. Do something about fluid retention before it causes bad temper, which could encourage you to quit trying to get out of your double trap.

If you seem particularly affected by sharp drops in your blood sugar, you should consider going all the way and "decaffeinating" yourself entirely. Use decaffeinated coffee or cola, or try Postum. If you don't expect it to taste like coffee, it's great. And finally, if weight gain is a consideration, here's another well kept secret: Caffeine is an appetite stimulant!

Caffeine takes you up and down hard and fast. You'll feel better without it, more alive and peppy, actually.

I want to repeat this: If you're quitting smoking now, and drink more than four cups of coffee or tea or three cans of cola a day, don't try to break your caffeine habit at this time. It's too much to demand of your body. Go slowly. Be kind to your body—it's the only one you have.

If, after you quit smoking and you want my help in gently breaking free of caffeine, refer to page 240 for information about CaffeinEnders.

10

What Do You Say to Someone You Love Who Smokes?

(And How to Help Your Child Say NO to Cigarettes—Even If You Smoke)

Trying to help someone protect himself from disease by suggesting he quit smoking can boomerang. The scenario is not uncommon. Here are some typical scenes.

The Lindquists have been married for about twenty-five years. It has been a good marriage—they've grown together and raised fine children. Arthur manages the small plumbing firm his father started. He is involved in the Lions Club, with Sight Saving as his pet project. He's moved up from Tail Twister to President and has a reputation for being a great sport.

Recently, Art developed a morning cough. He gags and coughs until he turns purple. Clara was suspicious that smoking aggravates his cough and decided to speak to him about it.

"Arthur, why don't you stop smoking for a while, so you can recover from that cough?" she suggested casually one morning.

He was defensive. "That cough has nothing to do with my smoking. It's just the dampness at the shop. I've ordered a new ceiling heater which should take care of it."

The cough got worse, and Clara began worrying about it. She suggested Art see a doctor. He was adamant. "Nothing is wrong with me. I'm fit as a fiddle. Lots of people cough—nothing to be alarmed about," he said impatiently.

His attitude was uncharacteristic, and the more she observed Art, the more she worried and the more certain she was that smoking was to blame. One day she bought a filter kit at the drugstore. The counter display said it could help the user to quit smoking. So she sprang it on Art at suppertime.

He almost growled at her as he threw it into the wastebasket. "Who said I wanted to quit smoking?" he asked. "If I want to quit, I will. I can quit anytime I want to," he said.

Lately Clara has become sarcastic about Art's cough and his smoking. Frustrated, she resorts to comments like "Oh, yes, we know when Art's home. His cough can be heard clear to Columbus. But he doesn't care!" Or, "Well, Art's going to smoke himself to death and I'll be a rich widow." Or, "He just doesn't have the willpower, and he isn't man enough to admit it and go for help."

A rift has developed between them. Clara doesn't understand how it happened—and Art is relieved when Clara isn't around to nag him about his smoking. Lately he has stopped at the bar for longer and longer before coming home after work. It's a rotten impasse.

Here is another illustration:

Jeannie Richardson, an attractive sophomore at Cornell, has been a regular smoker for about four years—since she started senior high school.

Her father smokes. Her mother never did. Her older brother, a medical student and varsity tennis star, quit smoking in high school because of his tennis. Jeannie is strong-willed and determined to take her place in the business world. She doesn't like to be told what to do or to take second place in anything.

Jeannie's mother often expresses disappointment that Jeannie smokes. "When I was a young girl," she says, "it was considered unladylike for young ladies to smoke." To which Jeannie quickly responds, "Those days are gone forever, Mother. We've come a long way, baby," as she dramatically and ceremoniously lights up to prove her point. Or, under friendlier circumstances, Jeannie will say, "But, Mother, all the girls smoke now. It's not what it used to be. And it helps so much when I'm studying and am under pressure—or when I'm bored."

When Jeannie's father is bothered to see her smoke (for reasons he can't seem to articulate), Jeannie is quick to remind him that he smokes, so it can't be so bad or he'd quit.

Once he tried to make a bet with her to see if they'd both quit together, but Jeannie refused. "You should be able to quit by yourself, Dad, because you've smoked a longer time than I. I enjoy smoking and want to go on until I'm closer to the time when it might hurt me. Then I'll quit."

When her father asked how she'd be smart enough to know in advance when it would be harmful, she said, "Well, I won't quite know in *advance,* but the minute the doctor tells me to quit, I'll quit."

Jeannie's father was defenseless. That was the reasoning he'd been using for the past twenty years. Lately he's worried; his doctor has told him to stop smoking because his breathing isn't what it should be for a man his age. There is a possibility of emphysema, the doctor has said. He has tried, secretly, to quit. But the more he worries about his health, the more he seems to want to smoke.

How can he tell Jeannie that it doesn't quite work the way she thinks it will? That once you're told "You must stop smoking," not only might it be too late, but it becomes unbearably difficult?

So what do you tell people you love who smoke? Obviously there are different answers depending on whether you want to protect children, whether you're a smoker yourself, whom you want to help.

First the no's:

1. Don't command them to stop smoking. Even if they're young, it's risky and often not successful. You're forcing them into opposition, forcing them to assert themselves.

2. Don't nag or harass. "Do you have to smoke another cigarette? You just put one out!" is perhaps the most common and most irritating comment to a smoker. Probably most used by nonsmoking parents to their children, it compels them to reinforce their position by thinking up new reasons why they need that next cigarette. You produce the same result by hiding their packs or yanking a cigarette from their hands. And don't think you're not nagging if you constantly clean up ashtrays after them. Even if you say you hate the smell of stale smoke and ash and you probably do—you're really saying you're a martyr to their smoking habit and want to make them uncomfortable. Remember what we said about martyrdom earlier on? It doesn't work.

3. Don't intimidate or demean by implying lack of character or willpower. Most smokers are aware that they shouldn't smoke; it's unfair, unkind and unproductive to bruise their egos. Don't criticize, and don't put up No Smoking signs, or you'll end up very lonely.

So what can you do to help someone come to terms with the smoking habit? Before I make some constructive suggestions, I'll tell you about the two events that affected me most in my struggle.

For years my family waged direct and open warfare on my smoking habit. It was too often the topic of conversation. And the more they'd hide my cigarettes, the more reinforced the habit became. Soon the very subject of smoking became an unpleasant one in our house. I would become defensive, my husband would become angry and the children felt helpless. Their helplessness and anguish proved to be a turning point in my attitude toward quitting.

One morning, our son Jim, then about eleven years old, came down for breakfast looking very pale and scared. I asked what was the matter, because he was generally a lively, happy boy.

"Oh, Mother," he said, "I had a nightmare. It was awful. I don't even want to think about it anymore, but I can't get it out of my mind."

"Tell me about it, Jim, and maybe it'll help to get it into the sunlight," I suggested.

"I dreamt we were at a place where there was a big wire fence, like the one around Grumman Aircraft on Long Island that we pass on the way to East Marion. It was taller than a person and seemed to be endless. Growing on this fence was a vine with big, shiny leaves. The vine was all over the fence as far as I could see. And on top of each section of fence there were signs. Big red signs, with neon lights blinking on and off.''

He was showing terror even as he spoke, reliving his dream. He was trembling and on the brink of tears. But he went on. ''The signs said, 'Warning. Do not touch these vines. Deadly poisonous upon contact.' ''

He couldn't seem to bring himself to finish. So I waited a moment and then tried to help him.

''And did you see yourself touching them, somehow, Jim, and that's what terrified you?'' I asked.

He started to cry, and sobbing, said, ''No, Mom, it was you! You had a basket, and you were picking the leaves and singing and saying how beautiful they were. When I tried to pull you away, and tried to show you the signs and begged you to stop picking the leaves, you just smiled and said, 'Silly little boy, they won't hurt me—and they're so beautiful.' '' Now he was unable to continue.

And now I was shaken, too.

And then he said one more thing, which hit home.

''I don't want you to die, Mom . . . I'm scared. And— and—,'' his voice and eyes lowered, ''you didn't seem to care how I felt.''

I asked him if he had any idea what the dream meant, but at eleven one is not very sophisticated at dream interpretation. He said he didn't know, but it was horrible and he was scared.

I hugged him and assured him it was only a dream and that he shouldn't worry.

But I had felt the impact of his dream. It had given me a clear glimpse of the deep hurt I was causing my family by my cavalier attitude toward potential illness and premature death.

To have an insight is a powerful experience. Although it's rare to really see inside a situation, into yourself or into your behavior, it can, when it happens, unleash a tremendously strong, though latent, motivation.

Jim's dream unleashed in me a great desire to quit, but I

still had the obstacle of knowing how. Because I had been so unsuccessful in the past, I was unable to respond immediately to my heightened motivation. That's when the next event took place. Jon, in his wisdom, decided it was time to stop the talk and find a way to do something about the problem. So he said, "Jackie, I know you have tried to quit very sincerely in the past, and I realize now that the smoking habit is more complicated than I thought. I understand that before you're able to quit smoking you have a problem to solve. But I have a problem too as a result. My problem is that I have the responsibility to protect my family, and especially our children. It would be unforgivable if I didn't do everything in my power to see that our children have their mother for as long as they need her. And I anticipate the day when smoking will finally cut you down. What shall I tell our children as we stand at the graveside and they look up at me and say, 'But Daddy, why did you let Mommy smoke?' "

He paused. "If you can tell me what to say, I won't bother you again about your smoking."

Jon wasn't cornering me just to show how clever or superior he was; he had a plan.

So when I wailed, "Oh, Jon—I've tried so hard to quit, but I can't. I'm weak. I'm stupid. I'm rotten to do this to you all. But I *can't* quit smoking," he had an answer.

"Yes, I know the problem," he said, "and I've done something about it. I have told the children the only way we could help Mother work out her problem was to give her the opportunity to really study the whole business of smoking and quitting. To give her time to research and work on the problem thoroughly, we would have to help with her daily chores like the laundry, grocery shopping and the cooking and cleaning.

"I asked them if they'd be willing to pitch in, if you'd be willing to give it a try," he added, "and they were enthusiastic."

This was an offer I couldn't refuse, because it was made in such an understanding way. And it was a positive suggestion, not an intimidating command.

The rest of the story is history. I did my research. The family did the chores. I worked out a method with which I could succeed and which left me with a feeling of personal freedom and enjoyment of not-smoking. And here I am, years later, writing a book to try and pass on what I've learned.

Here are my suggestions for helping others effectively:

What do you tell a youngster you love who smokes? Obviously, the problem is touchy. Young people are very much involved with the development of their own popularity, money and their image of themselves. One reason they may have begun to smoke was to challenge authority; for many of us smokers it was a rite of growing up. So you can explain that smoking is dangerous, but that may only make it more attractive: high-risk, glamorous, grown-up.

A spontaneous discussion can work, especially if it takes place with a slightly older peer who may have quit smoking because "it was kid stuff!" But obviously you can't count on that.

A wry aside came from my son Peter, who, when he was fifteen, wrote from school about being an overnight guest of a friend's. His young hostess, a smoker, was very much worried about her father's heavy smoking. "I spoke to one of her friends who says that smoking is uncool past about eighth grade, and she feels there's nothing wrong with not smoking."

I had to read it again: "Smoking is uncool past eighth grade." If that's where it's at with the young generation, I'm hopeful. But it's not always that easy. I've worked with students thirteen years old who had smoked for five years and were unable to quit without a program. They were as hooked as adults who had smoked for thirty years. Some of them wanted to quit and did.

If the "kid stuff" doesn't work directly, you will have to find a more subtle lure. "I'll have confidence that you can control your behavior and let you go hiking in Europe (or whatever the project is) if you can demonstrate that you're mature enough to stop smoking."

If you smoke or use "spit-tobacco," and have young children who have not yet started to experiment with tobacco—or a child who does—here's what you can do:

First, during a relaxed, loving time, open the topic, casually. Discuss your feelings; express your real concern about giving him/her the best chance to grow up healthy.

Then, because it's unprofitable to say to a child, "Do as I say, not as I do," tell them you're sorry you ever started smoking. When you did start, it wasn't known that tobacco caused serious health problem *and* you didn't know they were *addictive*. Now you are trying to quit (you are, or you wouldn't be reading this book), but it isn't easy because you're "hooked"—addicted. Tell them how you felt when you tried to quit in the past. The physical discomfort. The staggering realization that you weren't in control—that tobacco was.

That's why, if they smoke, you hope they will stop before it's too late, and if they haven't started, you don't want them to have to suffer and struggle to get free of it.

Mention that you feel that smoking has taken away a lot from you—including vitality, mental acuity, limits on sports participation, and MONEY! Calculate the amount you've smoked since you started, and the average cost per pack. (See "Cost of Smoking" charts and information in Appendices.) Tell your children what you might have used that money for—and then spend some time calculating what it would cost them if they start or continue to smoke.

I'm not a fan of bribery, but in this case it may have merit. Make a deal: "If you don't start smoking until you're twenty-one [statistics indicate that people rarely start smoking after twenty-one], I'll put $_ away each month and, with _% interest until you're twenty-two, it will compound to $_. If you don't start, or if you quit now, I'll pay for X." (Decide what they would like now—but keep it open for something they may want at twenty-two.) "However, if you start to smoke at any time between now and twenty-one, it's off. I'll go on a round-the-world trip. . . ."

You and your child should engage in this discussion fully. If the child is younger than around fifteen, it might be better to go for shorter times—and more age-appropriate bribes.

Remember, cigarettes are the "Gateway" drug. If you can prevent your child from starting to smoke, you have gone a long way toward preventing them from experimenting with alcohol, marijuana and other drugs.

This exercise assumes that you have enough ego strength to admit to your children that you have a frailty. That you made a bad choice as a youngster. And that you're sorry about it.

Also from the Surgeon General's 1988 report: ". . . we must take steps to prevent young people from beginning to smoke. First, we must insure that every child in every school in this country is educated as to the health risks and the addictive nature of tobacco use. Second, warning labels regarding the addictive nature of tobacco should be required for all tobacco packages and advertisements. Finally, parents and other role models should discourage smoking and other forms of tobacco use among young people. *Parents who quit set an example for their children.*"

Good news: As of January 1995, smoking will be prohibited in all facilities (that receive federal funds—that's almost 100%) where children under eighteen obtain services. That includes schools, libraries, day care establishments, etc. This is under the "Pro-Children Act" of 1994. The fine is $1000 *per* violation *per day*! The law includes faculty lounges, as well. Teachers will help, now, by setting a good example.

I feel this is a major turning point in the war to cut off the supply of new smokers—our children.

From the *New England Journal of Medicine*, 2/3/94, Herbert Kleber, M.D., Medical Director of CASA, Center on Addiction and Substance Abuse, Columbia University, "The legal availability of tobacco and alcohol for use by adults and the corresponding social attitudes about the use of these substances make it much more difficult to prevent their use by adolescents."

Regarding the issue of legalizing marijuana and other drugs, Dr. Kleber adds, ". . . it is likely to lead to substantial, even explosive use of drugs and be harder to turn around." Instead of legalization he believes more emphasis on treatment and prevention is required.

If you can prevent your youngster from starting to use tobacco, you will have acted to stem the use of all drugs.

Regarding legalization, I am very concerned that, unless marketing is completely controlled, it will be promoted as vigorously as cigarettes, and be used by more people—especially children—than otherwise. Obviously I am against opening that door. We are having enough trouble trying to put the cigarette genie back in the bottle.

WHAT CAN YOU DO?

1. Call or write your congressperson and senators.

Urge them to restrict young people's access to cigarettes. Ban vending machines. It is reported that children (under eighteen) bought 450,000 packs of cigarettes *a day* in 1990!

Urge them to increase treatment and prevention for tobacco, drug and alcohol use by children. Express your desire to have the cigarette tax raised substantially to support treatment and prevention through good educational programs and paid media advertisements to counteract the years of cigarette advertising. Remember, as I mentioned before: Cigarettes are the gateway drug. (As for funding: here are the staggering figures: There are presently fifty million smokers in the U.S. The average is one and a half packs per day. So if the tax is a dollar per pack, here's how that works out:

$$
\begin{array}{rl}
50{,}000{,}000 & \text{smokers} \\
\times\ 1\tfrac{1}{2} & \text{packs per day} \\
\hline
75{,}000{,}000 & \text{packs bought per day} \\
\times\ \$1.00 & \text{per pack tax} \\
\hline
\$75{,}000{,}000 & \text{(million) tax collected each day.} \\
\times\ 365 & \text{days per year} \\
\hline
\$27{,}375{,}000{,}000 & \text{(that's BILLION) a year.}
\end{array}
$$

That would pay for a lot of treatment and great ads. As for prevention, as the cost goes up, use goes down—especially among children who can't afford it.

Urge them to have nicotine levels printed on all packages of cigarettes, and a larger, bolder warning box, with the warning that "Nicotine is Addictive" printed ten times more often than each of the other warnings.

2. Discuss the need of the tobacco companies to recruit your child: In 1992 the average per capita number of cigarettes smoked in this country was 2,724 per day—if everyone over eighteen smoked. Each smoker that quits or dies means the tobacco industry must replace him or her with a NEW smoker. The only NEW smokers are children, since almost no one starts smoking over twenty-one years of age. So the cigarette companies NEED YOUR CHILD, and will do

everything in their power to seduce him or her. (See further about Joe Camel.)

3. On occasion, talk about the beauty and wonder of the human mind—and how delicately it is balanced. Your observations that it's rotten to have one's head disturbed— that thinking clearly, being able to reason and converse, and create, can be lost easily. Don't fool with your head. Drugs—beginning with tobacco—affect your head.

4. For younger children, play games parodying cigarette ads. Change the words to change the meaning or appearance. See Chapter 8 for other ideas.

5. Tell them about other kids who smoke: Seventy percent say they regretted starting smoking—didn't believe they would get hooked. Fifty percent say they have tried to quit, but can't.

6. If someone they know becomes hospitalized—or dies from a cigarette-related illness, discuss the cause, sympathetically. (I hope you have quit by this time, otherwise your child will be worried about you.) Sometime later, you can recite the facts: Smoking kills over 400,000 Americans a year. That's 1,100 a day. More than alcohol, fires, automobile accidents and AIDS combined.

7. Here's one that worked for many old-timers; it may or may not be a good idea for your young child. I wouldn't try it on a child fourteen or more—it could backfire. Buy a pack of high tar/high nicotine cigarettes. Considering that the lowest tar and nicotine brands have less than 0.5 mg of tar and less than 0.05 mg of nicotine, you should buy one of the following. The nicotine is very high—it causes nausea, lightheadedness, headache, stomachache and so on; the high tar causes painful coughing. (Can you do this to your beloved child?) When you offer to let them try smoking, tell them the rules: They must smoke a whole cigarette to the end— about ten puffs. They must inhale deeply after the first two to three puffs.

If they don't do this, they might start with low-tar/nicotine cigarettes, which make it much easier to start.

Following are the biggest, baddest . . . They are specific: size, filter, package. There are many levels of strength in each brand. Some are milder. These are highest in tar *and* nicotine:

Camel's 70 (length) non-filter soft pack	22mg tar	1.5 nic
Chesterfield King size, non-filter, soft	22mg tar	1.5 nic
Kool Reg size, non-filter, soft, menthol	21mg tar	1.3 nic
Luckies Reg size, non-filter, soft pack	25mg tar	1.6 nic
Pall Mall King size, non-filter, soft	26mg tar	1.8 nic
Phillip Morris, King, non-filter, soft	27mg tar	1.7 nic
Raleigh, Reg, non-filter, soft pack	23mg tar	1.4 nic

(From Federal Trade Commission Tar & Nicotine Report, 1993)

Since tar and nicotine levels change since FTC tests, check the cartons for the current tar and nicotine rating before purchasing one pack. Packs don't show the ratings.

8. Help your child avoid the physical causes of feeling "lousy," and, as a result, finding tobacco useful for the short-lived "lift" it gives. Reasons for feeling physically rotten are:

Tiredness, peplessness, grouchiness: make sure kids get enough sleep.

Acidity: Bad diet, stress: Drink milk to counteract the acid; for calmness.

Sugar: Even a little sugar causes a high and a subsequent fatigue. Help them cut down on sugary foods and drink.

9. PRAY!

Here are four key principles for reaching children, as determined by Americans for Nonsmokers Rights (ANR):

1. Young people are motivated to experiment with cigarettes because they believe it will increase their social status and because they believe that smoking is a way to mimic "adult only" behavior.

Your action: Teach kids that smoking isn't an adult behavior, but an addiction begun in childhood and most often continued unwillingly into adulthood.

2. Young people have a natural tendency to rebel.

Your action: Rebellion is a healthy phase of adolescent development. If teens need something to rebel against, direct their rebellion at the cigarette companies who use deceptive ads to trap kids into smoking.

Don't make being a non-smoker something that only "good" kids want to do, so that smoking remains a convenient way to rebel.

3. Young people need acceptance by their peers.

Your action: "Just Say NO" asks kids to turn away from peer pressure. It reinforces the message that peers want them to smoke. Strive to convince kids that being a non-smoker is cool. For example, teaching about *secondhand smoke* not only educates them about the harmful effects of environmental tobacco smoke, but also conveys the potent "smoking is socially undesirable" message.

4. Young people want to make their own decisions. They don't like being told what to do.

Your action: First show youth how the tobacco companies are trying to manipulate them. Second, contrast *free choice* with the reality of *addiction*. If they don't want their parents or teachers bossing them around, why let a pack of cigarettes do the same? Last, and most important, enlist their help in fighting tobacco and encourage them to create their own anti-tobacco activities.

In short, *empower youth to help themselves,* rather than dictate the anti-tobacco message.

The following blurbs are from the best book I have seen for kids—and adults: *Kids Say Don't Smoke*, text by Andrew Tobias, published by Workman Publishing, New York. $5.95.

It contains full-color posters by children, selected from more than 100,000 entries from 700 New York City schools. Each one chosen for the book is a contest winner. Each entry says, in its own way, "Don't Smoke." And the grown-up facts are eloquently compiled by Andrew Tobias, the financial wizard. It's the very best of what must be said to kids, their peers, and their parents. All royalties from the sale of the book go to Smoke-Free Educational Services:

> It's hard to get children to say NO to nicotine when the tobacco industry is spending $3 *billion* a year to get them to say YES.
>
> —Joe Tye, Stop Teenage Addiction to Tobacco (STAT)

The tobacco industry's argument that their $3 BILLION a year advertising budget isn't aimed at hooking new smokers—just persuading existing ones to switch is ludicrous. Emerson Foote, a distinguished humanitarian and founder of Foote, Cone and Belding Advertising Agency, later Chairman of McCann-Erickson, one of the world's largest advertising agencies, said, "I am always amused by the suggestion that advertising, a function that has been shown to increase consumption of virtually every other product, somehow miraculously fails to work for tobacco products."

If your youngsters argue that cigarettes can't be so bad or the government would make them illegal, tell them that if cigarettes were just invented today, they would never be able to advertise or sell them: (1) Nicotine is a poison; (2) it's addictive; and (3) the product of its combustion kills innocent bystanders. When tobacco is used exactly as intended, it causes disease and premature death. The Food and Drug Administration and Environmental Protection Agency would prohibit the sale of tobacco—in any form, except as a pesticide. Nicotine is a wonderful bug killer.

Dick Gregory said, "Even if I did smoke, I wouldn't do it in front of anybody because I wouldn't want them to know how stupid I was."

Dave Barry said, "Today, lighting a cigarette in a restaurant is about as socially acceptable as wandering around spitting into people's salads."

In a *60 Minutes* interview, a Bear Stearns financial analyst called cigarettes a poison disguised as a consumer product. The next day he was fired.

Cancer is a communicable disease. You get it from tobacco companies.

Begin to teach political action: RJR Nabisco uses Joe Camel—a cartoon character—to attract young smokers. They make Oreo cookies. How about boycotting Oreo cookies to express your indignation.

Speaking of Joe Camel. Someone sent me a Joe Camel matchbook. While R.J. Reynolds, maker of Camel cigarettes, claims they don't use Joe Camel to attract kids, let me tell you what the matchbook says. The cover shows a picture of a camel's face. He's wearing dark glasses, a white T-shirt and some kind of jacket. His hand is the main thing. It's holding a cigarette. Behind him is a sign, "Joe's Place." Printed on the bottom: "There's something for everyone at Joe's." So open the matchbook. Inside is the most childish "game" imaginable. Is this something an adult would do? "Get everyone together at Joe's Place! Put together the correct five matchbooks to create the entire Joe's Place scene. Impress your friends. Have them framed." (Really. Just what a forty-year-old would do, don't you think?) Or, light your Camels with them. Then 5 boxes [1] [2] [3] [4] [5]. The 5 is darkened, so I guess that's the number of the scene.

The scene is on the back. Two girls with camel faces and one boy with a camel face. On a table in front of them are two open packs of cigarettes: One Special Camels, one regular Camels.

This is very clever, insidious marketing to kids. As an adult, you can make them aware of this and defuse it. Kids don't like to be manipulated or fooled.

What can you do to help someone you care about who smokes cigars, pipes or uses chewing tobacco (also referred to as "smokeless" tobacco, or "spit" tobacco)?

If they tell you it isn't harmful because they don't inhale, here's the truth, from the Surgeon General's report of 1988: "All tobacco products contain substantial amounts of nicotine. *Nicotine is absorbed readily from smokeless tobacco . . . pipes and cigars . . . in the mouth or nose.* Levels of nicotine in the blood are similar in magnitude in people using different forms of tobacco. Once in the blood stream, nicotine is rapidly distributed throughout the body."

So not only are they causing serious physical harm to themselves (and others with their side-stream smoke), but they are addicted. This is often hard to take for smokers who choose pipes and cigars. Usually pretty independent types.

Since nicotine is responsible for causing serious cardio-vascular problems—heart attacks and strokes—cigar and pipe smokers are really not "safe."

But because cigarettes have dominated the media, cigar, pipe and chewing tobacco users have felt "safe"—that their tobacco use was harmless.

Here's the bad news: As the late Dr. Alton Ochsner put it when asked if there was a difference in risk between cigarettes, cigars, pipes or chewing tobacco, "It's just a matter of choosing the site of your cancer or type of your coronary disease . . ."

Pipe and cigar smokers feel they don't have to worry about lung cancer because they don't inhale. But now, with evidence that secondhand smoke kills, new research will undoubtedly suggest that because cigar and pipe smokers inhale their own secondhand smoke—at a dangerous level—they are subject to lung problems in addition to those other problems common to pipes and cigars: high incidence of mouth, throat, larynx and esophageal cancer, as well as heart conditions.

Cigar smokers suffer an increase in kidney and bladder cancers because they swallow the "juice." It just settles there and irritates those organs.

It won't surprise anyone when research on pipes and cigars is sufficiently funded to learn there are other significant health problems associated with those forms of tobacco use.

Spit tobacco users, unfortunately on the rise among adolescent boys because of tobacco-chewing baseball players, are subject to all the problems that nicotine and the toxic chemicals accompanying the tobacco create; however, the incidence of oral cancer is extremely high. It kills very young and very fast!

Because nicotine is a poison, it constricts your blood vessels, elevates blood pressure, activates hormones such as insulin, and too many other reactions from ingesting a poison to mention here; heart disease, including serious circulatory problems, results.

The fact is: Tobacco, in any form, kills.

What can you do to help someone decide to quit smoking a pipe, cigar or chewing tobacco?

Sometimes giving them the facts—that it's not "safe" simply because it's not mentioned in the media—can begin the process.

Offering the book as a gift, and then saying, "If I can help you break this tough, old habit/addiction, please let me know. I'll be here for you." But try not to nag. Show your concern because you care for the person, as with the approach to cigarette smokers, above.

I know you feel a sense of urgency—to try to end this game of Russian Roulette—but heavy-handed pressuring is counterproductive. (How do you feel when some big bully tells you you can't do something? You might just do it because you were told you couldn't. It's human nature.)

Instead try some ego approaches: If it's your mate, mention that kissing isn't so nice when the breath is foul from smoke . . . or lovemaking is affected because of the stale smoke odor on the body and in the hair, etc.

A better approach is the positive one—but you must seek opportunities to say something like, "Oh, you smell so nice when you don't smoke. I love to be near you."

If you get a new car, tell your smoker that, although they can't distinguish odors and fragrances because their olfactory nerve (smeller) is paralyzed from smoking, you think they won't want to allow it to reek of stale smoke—like the old one. (After a person quits smoking, they are often embarrassed to realize that they, their car, and their home reeked of stale smoke.)

And, of course, this book will work for your cause. Just keep it in sight. Don't demand that your smoker read it. If you think there's a section that might be particularly interesting—relating to a conversation you're having—open it up.

Be loving and sympathetic. Your smoker is hooked—and didn't know they would be when they started.

And as you have seen from my own example, the greatest help is manifest understanding and encouragement. You can sympathize with the hardship even if you've never smoked yourself. Don't criticize the other person's crankiness and irritability, which you should recognize as withdrawal symptoms. Say instead, "I can't quite imagine what it's like, but I respect you for trying. I believe in you."

But if the smoker cannot be persuaded to make an attempt at quitting, all you can really say is "I realize smoking must be a very complex and deeply personal thing. I've come to recognize that it is *your* problem. I can't force you to quit, and I can't quit for you. I can only tell you that I love you and believe in you and that I wish you wouldn't smoke because I'm looking forward to having many happy, healthy years with you. But it's your life, and I know you'll do the right thing when you're ready. And because it's *your* problem, I'm not going to say any more about it. Tell me if I can be helpful in any way and I'll do my best.''

11

Hunches About Why
People Smoke

(Whether Smokers Are Different and Why
They Go On Smoking)

One of our more delightful SmokEnder graduates is Chandler Sterling, an Episcopal bishop. He puzzled over the phenomenon of his smoking, his previous failures and his reasons for starting to smoke in the first place. He had a lot to say about the fact that he knows that smoking contradicted his deeply felt belief that the body is the temple of the soul.

Bishop Sterling is an unusual man, with wide-ranging interests; a man of the world as well as of the spirit; and he has a keen sense of humor. He has written a book about hockey. He's a sensitive person who is deeply concerned with the individual's day-to-day response to life. He told me one day about a conclusion he'd come to after a great deal of thought.

He thinks that a lot of us start smoking because it's a form of "gleeful sinning."

That is rather profound in a simple way. And I can't disagree with him. It could be one of the reasons that people start. A lot of reasons have been well and often quoted. But I'm not really trying to find the reasons why people start or continue to smoke. I'm convinced that people smoke because they don't know how to quit, that they haven't been properly prepared. I have tried to find why some of us, many of whom tried when we were young, did *not* take it up. My files are full of interviews with people who do not smoke, never have smoked. Why didn't they pursue it after that first (necessary) try? Why didn't they subject themselves to the same demanding learning process we did: the dizziness, the gagging and coughing, the awkwardness of the whole ritual, the embarrassment when we tried it out in front of others and they laughed, the burning throat and eyes?

Why did some people, like my husband, try a cigarette now and then and then decide consciously that it was not for him? Here are some insights I am led to consider.

One large group felt it didn't do anything for them and even wondered why others put themselves to the cost and trouble. Another group felt it was kind of dirty and expensive, and that their parents didn't approve. Another group tried it and gave it up because of the physical discomfort. Another, rather unusual, group confessed they had tried and tried to take it up because they felt inferior in the army and in college or business as non-smokers. This group reported unusual difficulties in starting to smoke and never achieved their objective. One friend in Providence, Rhode Island, a successful businessman and scholar, the father of four daughters, confessed a particular conscious embarrassment when he was younger because he didn't feel like one of the guys.

He's one of the guys now. Recently he mentioned to me how delighted he was that he finally feels in the majority and doesn't have to apologize for not smoking. Here's a man who very much wanted to smoke but was somehow repelled from the practice.

I have some hunches about the difference between those of us who took up smoking and those who didn't. There are factors I suspect must come into play, and one of them is youngsters' feelings about themselves. For instance, if they were generally popular, together, talented or accomplished in a particular field such as drama, music, sports, scholastics; if they felt good about themselves; the chances were *somewhat* less that they would start to smoke. It's still true. And that's very reasonable. And understandable. Except it doesn't hold up across the board. There are a large number of people who were very unhappy with themselves as teens, had a poor regard for themselves, but didn't start smoking.

One of my hunches has to do with *body chemistry*. I call it the "salt-lick" theory. You remember learning that deer need salt and search for "salt licks," like the lichen on the shady side of the tree, around the moss. They know by instinct that they need salt. And they look for it. Nature provides them with a way of replacing a missing element. It's not a learned hunger; it satisfies the need. These deer didn't develop a taste for salty things by munching on potato chips and peanuts during childhood.

Translate that to smokers, and you may suspect that *some people smoke to make up a lack of something in their chemistry*. The hunch seems to hold up in practice. An important section of the SmokEnder program deals with fatigue and lack of energy and the use of cigarette smoking to elevate the blood sugar. Many SmokEnder graduates value that self-knowledge and say it helped them to kick the habit, to live at a fairly high energy level without cigarettes. It would be an interesting experiment to measure the blood-sugar level of teenagers, and perhaps their thyroid activity, and then, when they were about twenty-five, to see which ones were confirmed smokers. My hunch tells me that those with below-average blood sugar and/or thyroid activity would be found among the smokers. Nicotine elevates the blood-sugar level, and each cigarette is a boost—a boost with a real kicker for the beginning smoker especially. The boost diminishes over the years and eventually is only a flicker. By then it's become a different problem.

On the other hand, it must be true that there are *people who react badly to the chemicals in cigarettes,* who have a reaction similar to hay fever, perhaps even stronger.

Also, there must be something to be learned about *how*

people perceive taste—in this case, the taste of cigarettes. Discounting the fact that most ads importune us to believe that we smoke for the taste, that the taste is good, I don't believe cigarettes taste good to most smokers.

If, for beginners, the taste of the first few cigarettes is perceived as vile and bitter, it could account for their not being tempted to take up smoking. It must be admitted, however, that most of us who yielded to the lure, who overcame all the difficulty, would admit that the first cigarette didn't taste so wonderful. Just as those first cups of coffee were disappointing. But to perceive a taste as vile is far from finding it a disappointment.

My hunch picked up some steam with the discovery that if monosodium glutamate is taken during the day it can cause cigarettes to taste bitter in the evening. I've been unable to track the source of that finding, but in a random testing among friends, it appears to hold up.

So here's another surprise trick to help you observe your smoking and perhaps change some conditions. Use some MSG on your food at lunchtime and you'll cut down on your evening smoking. Try it (unless you're on a low sodium diet or sensitive to MSG); but be certain you don't feel obliged to stuff food into your mouth that night instead of those bitter-tasting cigarettes, or you'll have another problem.

If you're the sort of smoker who could simply throw his cigarettes away if he had enough reason, this might do the trick for you. Many smokers have quit because cigarettes didn't taste good anymore, and some people report that cigarettes suddenly started tasting awful. Here's the hunch. Could it be that something in their body chemistry has changed enough to affect their taste? This is supported by the reaction that many pregnant women have to cigarettes and coffee.

Ah, one could become philosophical, dig deeply into taste, as art students think about color. What is green? Do you see the same thing I see when I see green? Can you describe green to me? What is taste? When you taste something sweet, is it the same thing I call sweet?

These are some things I think bear looking at if we're going to find out why we smoke. The undertaking is not very scientific, but it may help us to think about the satisfactions and answered needs. If we can lay our finger on some of the causes of our smoking, we may be able to find less dangerous and costly alternatives.

It is *the need to feel good* that I think may be a central point in trying to manage the smoking problem. Many of us are often not quite up to par. We want to get things done but we don't quite have the pep. Our energy levels may fall below what it takes to keep abreast of our more energetic colleagues. It's a natural phenomenon: the energy level drops from time to time during each day until the body manufactures more blood sugar to keep up with demand.

When we're little, we take naps. As children, we're put to bed at an early hour. When we become teens, we're more or less on our own schedule. Does it seem farfetched to imagine that the incidence of "tiredness" and peplessness which usually occurs first during our teen years is due to insufficient sleep, as well as other natural changes which occur during adolescence? Could it be that one of the reasons kids take to cigarettes so young is that smoking gives them a physical as well as an emotional boost?

Supporting this hunch is another intriguing guess. Studies have demonstrated that the chance of youngsters' smoking is less if their parents don't smoke. The implication has usually been that example is the prime motivator. "If your parents smoke, the chances are that you will smoke because you see them doing it and it's an accepted behavior" is a commonly accepted theory of the researchers.

I suspect the cause is partly *genetic*. If both parents smoke, perhaps both parents have the same lack in their body chemistry, and their offspring may have inherited that lack.

Carrying this idea a bit further and considering other areas of excessive (compulsive) behavior, it has been established by research into alcoholism that the offspring of alcoholics are more likely to become alcoholic. This would seem to point in the direction of my hunch even more clearly than the cigarette example: it's much easier to see the abusive effects of alcoholic excess than of smoking. So, one might reason, if a youngster saw his family wrecked and his father/mother deteriorate as a result of drinking, he would avoid that trap. That's not the kind of acceptable example a son or daughter might mimic. And yet alcoholism is said to be handed down.

My theory that some of us need our salt lick still holds even with these examples considered. What is missing that drives a person to hunger for tobacco, alcohol or sweets? The hunch carries over into the tendency to obesity. It too appears to be "inherited," according to current theories, of which the most popular is that fat mothers cook and serve the same fattening foods and serve them in the same fattening quantities they eat. So we become fat because of our eating habits, it is said—habits we "inherited" from thoughtless mothers. Poor mothers: they're blamed for so much.

I submit that we cravers, whether we crave cigarettes, whiskey or candy, have something in common. We frequently *feel "lousy" and go in search of sugar or other carbohydrates*. Each of these culprits either has a high carbohydrate content or causes a swift elevation of the blood sugar.

Another hunch that has pressed itself on my consciousness since I began my original inquiry is becoming less foolish each year. That was my suspicion that there was a relationship between the *peculiar acidy feeling* I sometimes had and the amount of smoking I did. I recall vividly the feeling I almost always had when I'd settle down for a long trip by car or bus. I would characterize it as acid indigestion or heartburn, but I knew it wasn't. (I was an old pro at both these feelings, having endured them to a considerable degree during my four pregnancies.) It seems to me that it was a sense of a low-level acidity. Now, as I write this and try to describe it to you, I find I can reconstruct the feeling by thinking about biting into a lemon. My salivary glands start pumping, but more significantly, something in that area which I visualize as above my stomach and below my diaphragm gets queasy or sour. Nevertheless, it was important enough for me to recognize that I reached for a cigarette to quell that feeling. And sure enough, it changed the feeling for a while.

And then I observed that I had that same feeling in some other situations—not necessarily related situations, but generally stressful. The more the feeling persisted, the more I smoked.

Having observed this condition during my close observation of my own smoking patterns, I concluded that it might be useful to try a simple antacid medication to see if it would lesson the number of cigarettes I smoked. It did. When I wrote my own program for stopping smoking, it included a package of Tums. When the sensation of "watery acid" inside me occurred, I popped a Tum instead of a cigarette. I didn't understand why, but it worked.

Now, after years of observing other smokers and their high-smoking periods, it seems to me there's a relationship between those of us who produce considerable acid under stress (or because of stress) and those of us who become smokers. It would be terrific to be able to say, "People who have taken up smoking have a higher acid level (produced more acid) than people who don't take up smoking. And the more acid in the system, the more cigarettes are consumed." If this is a fact, and I have a strong hunch it is, then we can do a lot to prevent smokers from starting and aid those who have already started.

Youngsters' acid balance could be quite easily stablized. In fact, another of my hunches is that youngsters who continue to drink quantities of milk regularly are less likely to start smoking than those who have given up drinking milk at an early age. Milk is alkaline. The lime (calcium) in it can counterbalance the acid in one's system.

Dr. Stanley Schachter of Columbia University, whom I have already quoted, has indicated that tests reveal a high acid content in urine as a result of anxiety and stress. He discovered that smokers who were given mild acids in large doses smoked more over a period of days than comparable smokers who took bicarbonates to make their urine more alkaline. His tests also show that bicarbonates reduce smoking under stress.

Here's what you can do to benefit from this possible relationship:

1. Don't drink orange juice first thing in the morning on an empty stomach. Put something solid into your stomach before your morning juice like bread or crackers to absorb acid.

2. Reach for an antacid tablet instead of a cigarette when you feel acidy.

3. Reduce the amount of caffeinated beverages you drink, which are highly acid. Switch to bouillon, herbal tea or water from time to time.

4. Drink milk, especially before bedtime and when your "nerves" seem to be taut. This is not just an old wives' remedy; milk is really an "acid balancer."

Another hunch. We have a real need for *breathing satisfaction*. Think about it. We take breathing for granted, yet it isn't a wholly involuntary action, like the heartbeat. We control our breathing. It's true that we can't hold our breath for too long, but we can regulate how often and how shallowly or deeply we breathe. My hunch is that smokers, taking those regular and deep drags on cigarettes, satisfy a need to breathe deeply. Or indulge themselves in a satisfying feeling.

Smokers who quit cold-turkey, and I had observed this about myself when I quit cold-turkey, complain of lightheadedness. I have watched them sigh deeply, and frequently. They were hyperventilating, as I had done so often. We needed to "feel" ourselves breathing, I think. Deep breathing is essential to well-being.

Here's how you can satisfy that "breathing need" before you quit and use correct breathing as a tool *after* you quit:

1. Learn to breathe deeply without a cigarette. Before you quit, taking long, deep breaths may cause a coughing fit, but it will pass, and you'll experience a similar sense of satisfaction to the one you got from drawing on your cigarette. Next time, before you reach for a cigarette, take one of those long, deep breaths—mouth closed—right down to your toes. Hold it for a moment or two and then exhale slowly through your mouth.

2. After you quit, whenever the desire for a cigarette hits you, stop what you're doing and take a slow breath. In through the nose, out through the mouth. It's like smoking, only better. You don't cough.

3. Don't sigh, and don't overbreathe. It causes lightheadedness. It's a form of anesthesia (I used it for natural childbirth).

One last hunch. *I think there must be a relationship between a reduction in the amount we breathe after we stop smoking and a slowing down of our metabolism. It may account for why some people gain weight.* Oxygen fans the flames of the fire that burns up calories. If the flame burns slowly, calories are not consumed as rapidly. Perhaps when we smoke, the breathing that is involved fans the flames and causes our metabolic furnace to burn more vigorously. If this is the case it's another reason to take conscious good, long, satisfying deep breaths regularly. But be careful: take only two or three at a time, or you may fade out for a moment.

These are only hunches; they're not meant to pose as scientific wisdom. It may even be that they have merit but for the wrong reasons. But this much I know: I used them to help walk away from cigarettes. I don't smoke anymore. Think about using them. They can't do any harm, and at the least, they should be able to help you cut down. Then, when you're ready to quit, you'll be in gear to do it with grace and style.

12

It's a Matter of Attitude

Good Attitude = Good Results
Poor Attitude = Poor Results

Earl Nightingale

The Stopping-and-Starting Syndrome

"It's easy to quit smoking. I've done it thousands of times," Mark Twain said, and you've probably heard that quote a thousand times. Another you may not have heard before comes from the British magazine *Punch*. When the tobacco tax had once again been raised on Budget Day, *Punch* predicted, "All the people who gave up smoking last year will do so again this year."

Both quotes make the point very clearly.

Whether you're a "passive" quitter who vows, "I'll stop tomorrow" but never skips a cigarette or an active quitter like me—we've all given up smoking from time to time for various reasons. Sometimes we succeed for a few days, a few weeks, even months at a time, and then go back. We're start-and-stop quitters.

In the same category belong the quitting "due to circumstances beyond my control" types. Classic example: when we're really sick, perhaps in an oxygen tent after pneumonia or a heart attack, we can't and don't smoke, sometimes long enough to believe that we've licked the habit. After returning home, when we feel better, the first chance we get puts us right back on the regular pattern.

Why can't we stay away from cigarettes? One accusation is that we smokers have a death wish. That's nonsense. I assure you that even through all the years I smoked, I had a feisty love of life and everything about it. In any case, as we've read, all the recent studies show that most smokers would like to quit if they only knew how. There's no death wish there.

Then we're told we go back to smoking because we're neurotic. I don't believe that either. As I've pointed out before, I believe that we are neurotic *because* we smoke. Another explanation of our failures, one we begin to believe ourselves, is that we suffer from a peculiar lack of willpower. As start-and-stop quitters we learn to accept failure. The more often we go back to smoking, the more we lose confidence. Slowly the acceptance of that failure spills over into other aspects of our life, just as success does. We quit quitting—it's too humiliating.

Mark Twain didn't have to tell us *why* he quit a thousand times. It doesn't really matter. All smokers know all the reasons why they should quit. They try out different reasons for different occasions, hoping one will click. In that respect, we're all passive quitters: we expect the reason itself to carry the burden, do it for us. Look at the pneumonia patient. He may even have been ultimately grateful for a circumstance beyond his control that gave him a good head start. He had no intention to quit: he suspended the habit because of necessity.

As long as we don't organize ourselves to succeed, we wind up by putting the blame on the latest reason in the latest attempt. Then it isn't we who have failed: the reason for quitting wasn't good enough and it let us down. That makes us victims. Deprived of pleasure, we feel sorry for ourselves; we suffer. To relieve the suffering we turn back to an old ally which never lets us down: the smoking habit.

If this startles you, imagine yourself as a compulsive candy eater. The process of not quitting is exactly the same.

How to Combat Failure

At this point I recommend that you go back to Chapter 4 and study the list of reasons why you smoke. Remember how we'd discovered that most of the ways in which you use cigarettes are merely conditioned responses, connections to daily activities, only habits.

The real reason why we don't quit—why we cannot quit without proper preparation—is that we're so conditioned. The habit represents comfort and solace; rewards on big and little occasions; a buddy we can rely on; the only luxury we indulge. The "one more won't hurt" is the hedge.

So we're not just addicted to nicotine—we're mired in a habit, and we have to rationalize it.

Let's have some fun by substituting words. First, for "rationale" read "excuse" and you'll find that instead of addictive smokers we are addictive excuse finders. Sounds silly, doesn't it? If that's a habit, we definitely ought to break it. Then, substitute "routine" for habit. To break ourselves of anything implies an irreversible, imposed action, something we automatically resist. So instead of breaking a habit we now read:

Let's Change a Routine

Routines are part of our daily life. We follow any number of them, as they save us time and effort as we do our daily chores. We don't think about them until we get bored or until a different routine becomes more convenient. Think of any routine that you've changed now and then, such as the way you go to and from work, or how you organize your laundry day. For years you used to do the laundry on Mondays. Then something came up that could be done *only* on Mondays, something that made your life more interesting—a club meeting, a bridge party, a part-time job. So you moved the laundry to Tuesday. No problem. Or what about the Sunday-morning routine—whether to have a long bath or a leisurely breakfast first. When you felt there was an advantage in the new routine, it was a preference; it didn't require any willpower. In a previous chapter we called this rearranging priorities. It's more or less the same thing.

Willpower is an odd concept, one that is often both used and misused. Throughout this book I have tried to condition your mind toward a positive attitude, mostly in the way I've tried to use my own and other people's positive and forward-looking experiences to modify discouraging memories of struggles and failures. Stay with me while I explain the positive part in more detail.

The power of our will is the power of the "great human mind" which helps us to achieve the impossible. Sir Edmund Hillary used his willpower to reach the peak of Mt. Everest, after his mind had convinced him that that was what he wanted to do more than anything else. Willpower works to support our mind, though it may cause some pain and hurt when we're trying to force it. In fact, no amount of willpower can make us do something that we don't really want to do. But as soon as our mind starts to meet willpower even halfway, the struggle begins to diminish. Let's play around with this for a minute, and then you can carry the exercise as far as you want.

"I don't want to go out in this weather and trudge to the office, but I have to." That's a completely negative statement and makes you miserable. Now modify the statement by using different reasons. "I don't want to go out in this weather, but I have to or I will lose my job, and I need the money." Now your reluctance is somewhat diminished because you have plans for the money.

Now see how a different reason begins to change the way you formulate that same thought. "I hate to go to the office in this weather, but we have the important meeting today," or even, "but I'd rather go in today because I want to take Monday off." Your preferences are beginning to balance the negative and positive attitudes, and you have greatly reduced the willpower you need to make yourself go out.

Then compare that with "Normally I wouldn't want to go out in this weather, but we have theater tickets for tonight and have waited weeks to see the play." No lack of willpower here; in fact, it would take willpower to keep you at home.

You can compose dozens of sentences like that. You can also make a sentence that goes "I don't want to give up smoking but I have to or I'll die."

We've discussed that argument before and found it wasn't convincing enough because we all have to die sometime. It's just too negative. But see how the meaning changes, and your attitude, too, if you add, ". . . before I've really lived," or ". . . before I see the children grown up," or whatever other wish you'd like a chance to fulfill.

What Can Make You Quit

It is my belief that you can free yourself of the smoking habit once you change the smoking routine by establishing other preferences for yourself.

Make the task easier. Establish a positive attitude for your reasons to quit—not as a form of self-denial or sacrifice, but as an exchange for something that's of greater value. That's an interesting twist, particularly when most smokers are used to thinking of quitting as giving up something they consider worthwhile.

Here's an amusing example of that sort of change in attitude—a true story. I was told of a man who had been a heavy smoker but had stopped at a time when TV cigarette advertising was still allowed. He remarked, "I was getting more and more annoyed by the stupid cigarette commercials. One day, when I was watching a particularly inane situation, I decided I wasn't going to support that kind of stupidity anymore. I stubbed out my cigarette and haven't smoked since."

A cigarette commercial that made him quit smoking. Funny? But, of course, his mind had subconsciously concluded that there were better uses for his body, money, time. It doesn't matter how much or how little of the reason was clear to him at the moment. The main thing is that his mind had found a better way, and he needed no willpower to exchange something that was no longer worthwhile for something he wanted more.

Dr. Donald T. Fredrickson, a pioneer in the smoking-cessation effort and now a dean at New York University, Post Graduate Medical School, puts it into more scientific language. As a member of the New York City Board of Health, Dr. Frederickson had the responsibility of providing citizens of New York City with a practical means of freeing themselves from the smoking habit. On the basis of his work at the clinics he had set up, he wrote his opinion of the key to lasting success: "As we see it, there are two attitude postures one can opt for during withdrawal. One is negative and basically self-defeating. The other is positive and can be powerfully self-reinforcing.

"When the smoker opts for the self-defeating attitude, he tends to view withdrawal as an exercise in self-denial . . . that an object of great value is being taken from him . . . one that may be a source of pleasure. . . .

"When a smoker opts for the positive, self-reinforcing posture, he looks upon withdrawal as an exercise in self-mastery. Rather than taking something away, he is adding to his life a new dimension . . . bringing in turn a renewed sense of one's ability."

It happened to me. It's happened to many others. In fact, it is the very reason I am determined to spread the word, through the SmokEnder program and through this book. Not only is it possible to quit smoking without pain, but there is a mighty good chance that many other aspects of your life will be the better for it.

Here's one more example of how knowing your preferences can help you to stay an ex-smoker even when you're under stress. It happened to Barbara Davidson, now a fine Moderator in our program.

"One fall night," she says, "I checked in with my husband as I was leaving class. He reported that all was well at home and I said, in that case, I'd stop in at a neighbor's house on the way home to help plan the block association's annual children's Halloween party.

"About twenty minutes after I arrived at my neighbor's, I received a frightening phone call from my husband, who was at New York Hospital with our three-year-old boy. They were pumping out his stomach! He had found a bottle of Vicks Vapor Steam and had drunk it down. Camphor, the main ingredient, is highly poisonous. I dashed out of my friend's home and hailed a taxi, my heart pounding audibly. I screamed at the driver to get me to the hospital, that it was a matter of life and death.

"He responded to my panic by nervously lighting a cigarette and took off like a shot. I thought I need one too. This is the worst thing that has ever happened to me. Just as I was ready to ask the driver for a cigarette, I remembered what we had learned at SmokEnders: smoking never makes anything better. What was it that I really wanted?

"1. I wanted the taxicab to go faster. Where had all this traffic come from?
2. I wanted to be told my son was going to be all right, that he would live and not suffer any permanent ill effects.
3. I wanted to put my arms around my child and feel him breathing, hug and kiss him, and take him home.
4. I wanted my husband to put his arms around me and tell me not to worry.

"It was very simple. Once I knew what I really wanted, I could see that it wasn't a cigarette."

When we hurt inside, it's an emotional discomfort. As smokers, we condition ourselves to believe that lighting up relieves us of even those things which weigh heavy on our hearts and minds. It never does, of course. The problems are there long after the cigarette has been put out. It's important to try to articulate what you want. Once the real thoughts are permitted to take shape in our mind, you can see that you don't want a cigarette. You want the problem, the pain, a situation, fear, anger, hurt to go away. This is a good thing to know. It's like having a secret weapon.

Bridging the Gap

You may remember that I told you in "A Personal Note from Jackie Rogers" in the beginning of the book that my main reason for writing it was to help you cross the span between deciding to quit and making it stick. If you don't remember, or if you didn't read it, go back to it now. It was my intention to start you off with all the good, positive and joyful lessons I learned and to share them with you. I've touched on them in almost every chapter, but now I'll put all the steps together.

1. Know yourself. Face up squarely to why you smoke,

how much smoking really means to you and why you'd like to quit.

2. Don't be afraid that it's too late. It was a turning point in my attitude when I came to realize, and could state with conviction, that *my body would restore itself*. And it did. Quickly.

3. Learn to decide when you really want to quit and when you're only suspending the habit. That's very important. There's nothing wrong in itself with just suspending. At the very least, it will give your body a chance to recoup. Thousands of people give up smoking for Lent without too much trouble. They know it is only an interlude, and that knowledge sustains them. Once you have found you can stop for a limited time, you may find it easier to go the whole day. It's part of getting ready.

4. Once you really want to be serious, use the best reasons you've come up with to adapt your own attitudes. Set yourself a goal that's worth the trouble and keep it in front of your mind. My favorite example of that is what I call the De Gaulle method. As I remember hearing it, General Charles de Gaulle declared to his staff one day during the early years of the war, "I'm not going to smoke anymore," and being De Gaulle, he didn't. I don't remember whether we were told his reason, but it's conceivable that he finished the sentence "until France is free again." But regardless of whether it was a high ideal, sheer willpower or his ego that wouldn't allow him to back down, he suppressed his desire. No doubt he suffered from his craving, but he found other ways of refocusing his desire.

We ordinary people may not have quite such high ideals as the general's to sustain us. Happily, you don't need the willpower of a De Gaulle to stop smoking. You can do it much more easily this way.

5. In the SmokEnder program, we spend considerable time training smokers in the art of distraction. Reshape and reorganize your habits by changing your rewards systems. Instead of reaching for a cigarette, *reward yourself* by "goofing off" for ten minutes and doing something completely different. Something you know you shouldn't be doing at the time but that gives you pleasure. It interrupts the pressure of the moment and reduces the need to smoke.

6. Above all, learn to walk away from self-pity. Develop a sense of humor. Look at yourself the next time you feel self-pity starting to flow. As an amused parent would watch a loved child, smile at yourself and say, "That kind of feeling is kid stuff, and I'm grown up now. Self-pity is childish; it's not to be taken seriously anymore."

In the SmokEnder program we found that a number of those who had previously failed had not fully understood the way self-pity works in us. They had paid scant attention to understanding themselves and weren't even aware that they had a habit of feeling sorry for themselves. But believe me, *one of the biggest reasons we smoke is because we need the recognition, reward and comfort that we've come to believe smoking stands in for.* And *the biggest reason we fail is that we have been conditioned to believe that giving up smoking is a form of sacrifice.* But we know better now!

These are really the basic mental and emotional points you need to observe in order to succeed. They are intensely practical; there's nothing mysterious about them. As I mentioned earlier, William James, the father of modern psychology, studied habit formation and came to recognize the essentials of making or breaking a habit. He wrapped it all up in a few sentences. You must first convince yourself that the new habit has value for you; then you must lay out a plan and practice it without exception. "Never suffer an exception," he said. And finally, once the new attitude is developed, you must never again "feed" the old habit.

There's one major point to consider before you can proceed to the actual quitting process: Motivation.

13

Motivation: the Key
(What's in It for Me?)

"**W**hat's in it for me?" you might ask, correctly. Perhaps you wonder if you're ready to confront quitting head on. It's a question of priorities. You've had a chance to look deeply into yourself, have discovered that you are the most important person in the world; you like yourself, and you care enough about your life to want to live it to your fullest potential. That's a good start.

Perhaps you were told you ought to quit smoking by your doctor. Perhaps a doctor or loved one even read you the riot act and said you had to quit smoking or else. Maybe that even scared you into a few weeks or months of abstinence and you went back as soon as the scare wore off, rebuilt your wall of rationalizations.

Have you ever quit smoking because you *wanted* to—from strong personal desire, pure and simple? Did you ever quit because the "want to" rather than the "have to" or "ought to" prevailed?

"Why should I want to?" Perhaps the burdens of smoking are becoming too numerous. The indignities, both physical and psychological, that you have sustained make you angry. Even better, perhaps the benefits are becoming irresistible. Graduates often tell me how amazed they are by the mighty accumulation of "pluses" they experienced when they quit smoking.

Here is a quiz to determine whether there's enough value in it for you finally to consider a serious attempt at quitting smoking.

I have discovered in my work with smokers that the benefits can be broken down into three basic categories: Physical, Emotional and Social. Here are *one hundred sixty* benefits. They were expressed by SmokEnder graduates after just four weeks of not smoking.

BENEFITS OF QUITTING

These statements are authentic; the names of the ex-smokers who made them are on file. They are real people, like you.

As you read the list, ask yourself if each item would be a benefit to you. To what degree? Circle the letter—A, B, C, D or E—that defines the degree.

I'm not going to include the most obvious benefits, such as "I've reduced my chances of getting lung cancer and heart disease . . . I won't suffer from emphysema . . . I'll never have Buerger's disease; I'll have good health" . . . Good health so you can do what? Live longer. Why? The benefits listed below are smaller and all concrete. They are about, as we often say at SmokEnders, the quality of life and the enhancement of ego.

> A—Has no significance for me at all
> B—Slight interest to me
> C—It would be helpful
> D—Sounds very good to me
> E—Galvanizing!

Don't skip. It is important that you respond to each suggestion. Ask yourself, "Would I be happy to make that statement?'' Then recheck the list and you'll see *your* reasons for wanting to quit. The D and E column will show you *what's in it for you to quit smoking*.

PHYSICAL BENEFITS

(CIRCLE ONE)

1. I never realized I could have so much energy. A B C D E
2. My sense of smell has improved considerably. A B C D E
3. I have a general feeling of well-being and feel more fit. A B C D E
4. No short-windedness, and I'm breathing easier. A B C D E
5. Mouth is no longer dry; tongue is no longer "brown." A B C D E
6. Eyes are bright and clear, no longer bloodshot or puffy. A B C D E
7. It's easy to ride my bike now—even up hills. A B C D E
8. I can't believe it, but I'm no longer craving nicotine or climbing walls. A B C D E
9. Sore throat is completely gone. A B C D E
10. Smoker's cough is gone. A B C D E
11. Breath smells fresh and clean and my mouth tastes better. A B C D E
12. Find I have more time to do things. A B C D E
13. Foods and drinks have sharper, clearer tastes. A B C D E
14. Had a facial today—now maybe my face will stay cleaner. A B C D E
15. Can breathe through my nose now instead of my mouth for the first time in years. A B C D E
16. Nasal passages are free from burning and no longer congested. A B C D E
17. My hair stays cleaner longer and doesn't stink of smoke. A B C D E
18. Find I can climb stairs easily *and* talk at the same time; delighted not to have to stop at every landing to "admire the view." A B C D E
19. Housework doesn't fatigue me anymore. A B C D E
20. Beginning to feel alive again. A B C D E
21. Don't feel "down" before I get up in the morning. A B C D E
22. Fall asleep more easily and wake up refreshed. A B C D E
23. No more heart palpitations. A B C D E

24. Can swim better than in years—continuous laps, and even once across the pool underwater. A B C D E
25. Feel calm. A B C D E
26. No pain in my chest anymore—can even laugh at a joke without it hurting down there. A B C D E
27. Played two sets of tennis and my legs finally tired before my wind ever did. A B C D E
28. I don't smell like stale smoke; I don't taste like stale smoke. A B C D E
29. More feeling in toes—went for a walk in freezing weather and my toes and fingertips didn't hurt from the cold. A B C D E
30. No more black sputum coming up. A B C D E
31. I no longer bulge in strange places from boxes of cigarettes stashed in various pockets. A B C D E
32. Don't have to sit in smelly smoking sections of movies, airplanes, commuter trains; have freedom of choice, rather than being "banished." A B C D E
33. House is definitely cleaner. A B C D E
34. No need to keep emptying ashtrays; saves time and energy. A B C D E
35. Acid indigestion is gone, and no more sour stomach. A B C D E
36. No more waking up in the middle of the night, and the attending "bladder condition" has disappeared. A B C D E
37. My skin looks alive, and the grayish-yellow pallor is gone. A B C D E
38. I enjoy looking younger and feeling younger. A B C D E
39. My hands no longer shake. A B C D E
40. No more black dots in front of my eyes. A B C D E
41. I'm dancing again—forgot how much fun it is. A B C D E
42. Began jogging daily—couldn't do this before for any period of time. A B C D E
43. Doing advanced yoga breathing daily. A B C D E
44. My walk seems to be more jaunty—purposely walking on sunny side of street so passersby can see how great I feel. A B C D E
45. I'm enjoying flavors and aroma I haven't experienced in years. A B C D E
46. I've cut down on coffee consumption—another addiction. A B C D E

47. No more of those late-afternoon headaches.   A B C D E
48. Have more vitality during the day.   A B C D E
49. Getting better at exercise; enjoying it more, too.   A B C D E
50. Sex hasn't been this good in a long time!   A B C D E

SOCIAL BENEFITS

51. I enjoy lots of good feedback from people I love.   A B C D E
52. It's great to be able to make a point without waving a cigarette in your adversary's face.   A B C D E
53. No longer have to scout for ashtrays upon entering someone's home.   A B C D E
54. I enjoy not burning myself, my possessions, other people or their possessions.   A B C D E
55. No more excuses for myself to my family, my physician, my boss or my friends.   A B C D E
56. Glad to have eliminated a habit that today is considered socially offensive.   A B C D E
57. Don't have to carry cigarettes during a party; two hands free—one for drink, one for hors d'oeuvres.   A B C D E
58. Pleased with myself for being a trend setter—smoking is no longer "in."   A B C D E
59. No longer late for appointments because of running back into the house to see if I "left one burning."   A B C D E
60. My date didn't have to keep waving smoke away all evening.   A B C D E
61. Am appreciative of good cooking—no longer have to rush through the meal to light up.   A B C D E
62. Was finally able to venture an opinion on some vintage wine without being told, "How would you know? Smokers can't taste anything."   A B C D E
63. No longer will I make a fool out of myself cursing out delinquent cigarette-vending machines that "don't deliver."   A B C D E
64. No longer so clumsy now that I have an extra hand.   A B C D E
65. Didn't have to smell up my friend's apartment.   A B C D E

66. Was able to break a child's fall without fear of singeing him.   A B C D E

67. Easier to get close to people without having to worry about smoker's breath or smoker's odor.   A B C D E

68. Was able to beat someone at tennis who is ten years younger than I am!   A B C D E

69. Clothes smell fresh, stay cleaner longer.   A B C D E

70. Feel at ease with people.   A B C D E

71. Don't have to sit apart from people to accommodate my ashtray, smoke clouds, etc.   A B C D E

72. Can enjoy theater without getting impatient for the intermission.   A B C D E

73. Have been told I'm more "kissable."   A B C D E

74. Fellow taxpayers and insurance-policy holders will not have to bear the financial brunt of my smoking-induced diseases.   A B C D E

75. The social "crutch" is not needed anymore.   A B C D E

76. I don't hide behind a cigarette.   A B C D E

77. Sat through a really great movie, twice, and never thought of a cigarette.   A B C D E

78. Cocktail before dinner no longer a trigger; nor wine with the meal.   A B C D E

79. Never dreamed I'd be an inspiration to others.   A B C D E

80. Didn't volunteer myself into a lot of "sorry situations" with great potential for self-pity, poor-me reactions.   A B C D E

81. Feel more poised in social situations.   A B C D E

82. Not reluctant about being physically close to others, as I think I smell good.   A B C D E

83. No more anxiety about dropping ashes in other people's homes or begging for an ashtray.   A B C D E

84. Believe it adds to my salesmanship not to have to subject customers to smoky rooms.   A B C D E

85. I'm encouraging others to stop smoking; I guess that makes me a trend setter.   A B C D E

86. Everyone around me seems delighted that I do not smoke; one might say that I'm (you should pardon the pun) de-lighted too!   A B C D E

87. Smoking is aesthetically ugly.   A B C D E

88. Am more talkative, not as shy.   A B C D E

89. No longer seen as an addict.   A B C D E

90. Don't have to excuse myself anymore to "run out" for a pack.   A B C D E

91. Don't have to fear burning loved ones or
myself.   A B C D E
92. I no longer impose my smoke on hapless
victims.   A B C D E
93. Feel more like everyone else now, sort of
normal.   A B C D E
94. Can concentrate on other people's
conversation—I listen better without the
distraction of a cigarette.   A B C D E
95. People don't complain or give me angry looks
about polluting the air.   A B C D E
96. When I shop at the department store, I don't
have to stand in that smoky, oppressive
vestibule between the two sets of glass doors,
finishing my cigarette on the way in . . .
lighting up on the way out.   A B C D E
97. Love carrying a small evening purse . . . used
to need a larger one to accommodate all my
smoking paraphernalia.   A B C D E
98. Won't ever burn anyone else again in an
elevator.   A B C D E
99. Co-workers are so very supportive, and so
many compliments on my success.   A B C D E
100. I'm no longer discriminated against.   A B C D E
101. Love life has definitely improved!

EMOTIONAL BENEFITS

102. I enjoy increased self-confidence.   A B C D E
103. I have tremendous feelings of
accomplishment and pride.   A B C D E
104. It's great to be able to deal with stressful
situations calmly and maturely.   A B C D E
105. The "no concessions," can-do attitude is
spreading to other areas of my life.   A B C D E
106. Tremendous self-esteem which allows self-
respect to return.   A B C D E
107. I love being able to "get to things" right away
instead of wasting five or ten minutes finishing
a cigarette.   A B C D E
108. Such great feelings that come from having
done something positive and very special for
me, myself.   A B C D E
109. Wonderful not to need to buy cigarettes, not
to have to carry them around, not to have to
worry if I left them somewhere.   A B C D E

110. It's great to know that I can cope with
anything now that I've quit smoking.   A B C D E
111. I enjoy having more money.   A B C D E
112. What a relief not to have to worry about
starting a fire by accident.   A B C D E
113. Feel so proud of myself.   A B C D E
114. More in touch with my feelings.   A B C D E
115. Dealing with stress directly rather than
resorting to cigarettes.   A B C D E
116. Sense of well-being permeating everything.   A B C D E
117. Able to eliminate self-pity instead of
wallowing in it and smoking a lot.   A B C D E
118. I look in the mirror and see me smiling back.   A B C D E
119. I feel I've accomplished a fabulous task.   A B C D E
120. Happier, stronger, more relaxed and secure.   A B C D E
121. Don't need cigarettes to resolve my problems
and/or conflicts.   A B C D E
122. I feel like a winner!   A B C D E
123. Sense of power and self-mastery.   A B C D E
124. I "shape up" and face situations, rather than
erecting a smoke screen.   A B C D E
125. I guess I showed 'em!   A B C D E
126. No more guilt.   A B C D E
127. Beautiful sense of serenity.   A B C D E
128. I'm so happy.   A B C D E
129. My disposition seems to have improved; I
smile a lot more.   A B C D E
130. Looking forward to so many things; daring to
dream and plan again.   A B C D E
131. Don't need excuses anymore to leave the
house so I can smoke.   A B C D E
132. One less anxiety-producing thing to worry
about—panic is gone.   A B C D E
133. I've given my positive emotions to people and
to rewarding activities rather than to
cigarettes.   A B C D E
134. No longer have to make excuses for myself.   A B C D E
135. Peace of mind.   A B C D E
136. Sat in endless traffic, then waited in long line
at airport—both without that desire to smoke.   A B C D E
137. Gives me a feeling of getting a "new start"
in life.   A B C D E
138. I can say it: I don't smoke anymore!   A B C D E
139. Anxiety has changed into energy.   A B C D E
140. I don't have to be afraid anymore.   A B C D E

141. No longer have to make promises to myself
     that I will quit smoking.   A B C D E
142. If I can quit smoking, I can do anything!   A B C D E
143. Support from family and friends is rewarding. A B C D E
144. Feel like a celebrity—everyone asking me,
     How did you do it?   A B C D E
145. New dignity.   A B C D E
146. Feel relaxed in "no smoking" areas where
     once I would have felt personally threatened. A B C D E
147. No longer have to make excuses to my
     children.   A B C D E
148. The hysteria has gone out of my life.   A B C D E
149. Petty things that used to bug me don't even
     get a rise out of me anymore.   A B C D E
150. By quitting smoking I have proved to myself
     that I do take responsibility for my own
     behavior—for my own life. I'm no longer
     ashamed of me, but proud of the new mature
     me!   A B C D E
151. The feeling of self-mastery is thrilling. It
     eluded me for the past six years because I
     couldn't quit smoking.   A B C D E
152. How nice not to feel embarrassed. I feel like
     a first-class citizen again.   A B C D E
153. I'm Canadian. Cigarettes are six dollars a
     pack. My family and I are planning our dream
     trip to Alaska with the $2,200+ I'm going to
     save this year.   A B C D E
154.   A B C D E
155.   A B C D E
156.   A B C D E
157.   A B C D E
158.   A B C D E
159.   A B C D E
160.   A B C D E

(After you quit, add your reasons to this list.)

Here's What to Do:
Review the E Column. These are *your* reasons for wanting
to quit. Your Motivators. If you have less than five E's,
review the D list for those that inspire you. If you didn't
take time to thoughtfully read these reasons, please take
time now. It's important.

You will be asked to search more deeply for your own reasons in the weeks ahead, but for now:

1. In your notebook, write "Reasons I want to Quit" on top of a new page. Leave several blank pages following.
2. Start your list with the reasons you found on this list.

14

Now That You're Ready

(Get Set and GO)

Self-conquest is the greatest of victories.

—PLATO

NOTE: If you want the optimal chance for long-term success—and the easiest, most comfortable Cut-Off, please don't read this chapter until you have read through the rest of the book. The messages in the book—some subtle, some blatant—will affect your attitude about smoking and increase your motivation to quit so much that the following instructions will have additional power. Why take a chance on your success?

You deserve the best. You surely know there are many ways to quit smoking—some better than others. The important question you should ask is, "What is the quality of the quit?" Will you feel FREE and joyous—or will you fight the craving and sense of loss for years? Will you relapse easily or will you be physically and emotionally prepared to stay off tobacco forever? If you have read this book from the beginning and worked at the various "assignments" designed to engage your mind in this, you are properly motivated. You've begun the process. Now you're ready to take the habit apart, piece by piece, step by step, and emerge victorious.

Mark Twain (and I) said, quitting is easy. I've done it thousands of times. The goal is to shed the craving and all the triggers that are buried deep inside from decades of repetitive practice; shedding old belief systems; facing the reality of your own competence—and your vulnerability; and to grow up, that last little bit, so you stop feeling sorry for yourself as a victim.

It takes unlearning old practices, and relearning new ways. It takes a powerful change in attitude from "I can't" to "I can and I will." It takes letting go of an old "romance" with a mean-spirited lover: tobacco (it was ready to hit and run as soon as it made you so sick you couldn't smoke anymore), and then being glad that you broke up—instead of wishing you'd get back together again. It's a lot of buried and concealed actions, feelings, beliefs, and practices that you wove into a complex fabric of your smoking life.

Now you're ready to do it right. Your motivation is high. Take advantage of it. You're very likely excited about the possibility of quitting and think there might be something good in it for you. There is. Freedom and Self-Mastery are two of the most precious gifts you can give yourself. I received those gifts: freedom from craving and a wonderful boost in self-esteem. That's what I want to share with everyone.

Here's where you begin.

First, make a commitment to yourself that you will follow the instructions fully and enthusiastically. Do them as if your life depended upon it. It likely does.

Don't pick and choose. You may be highly educated and extremely competent, but in this matter, permit me to tell you, you are a novice.

An important suggestion worth repeating: Whenever you read something that really hits you, feel free to write in the book. Highlight words, paragraphs, sections or whatever. Dog-ear pages that you want to get back to quickly. Put Post-It notes in special places with your comments or insights on them.

Carry this book, your notebook, Hi-Liter, Post-It notes and a pencil with you everywhere. The book is your "coach"; your notebook will become your bible. You'll be glad you have them for a long time.

Where do you begin? You can either join SmokEnders if a seminar is within your area (check your telephone book, or call 1-800-828-4357) or you can make a commitment to yourself that you will follow these instructions fully and enthusiastically.

The SmokEnder program is a highly structured six-week seminar and builds on a number of crucial elements, such as your own personal involvement, accountability to someone each week, the play of dynamics among the entire group and, most especially, the personal guidance and understanding of a trained Moderator.

To date, the only means of presenting the method effectively is in the seminar framework, the Audiocassette Home Study Program, and this book. It would be wonderful if we could have seminars everywhere, but even then there are people who couldn't avail themselves of them. I wish we could put it into capsules or tablets and distribute them throughout the world as a sort of mass inoculation to quickly help all smokers who want to quit. That would be about 90% of all smokers, according to a recent report by the U.S. Department of Health and Human Services.*

Unfortunately, SmokEnder seminars are available only in large cities, except in corporate settings. That's why I wrote this book—to reach smokers everywhere in the world.

Note to Nicotine Replacement Users—Gum or Patch

If you're using this book to deal with the psychological aspect of your smoking problem, while the gum or patch deals with the physiological (addictive) aspect, here are a few special instructions.

Don't smoke while on nicotine replacement—ever. It could be fatal. So when the instructions for the regular program are to smoke, or monitor your smoking, simply observe the times you have the IMPULSE to smoke.

The Health Benefits of Smoking Cessation: Report of the Surgeon General. 1990.

Follow your physician's or dentist's orders exactly. Stay on at least ninety days—not longer—unless the doctor orders otherwise. Nicotine, taken into the body by any means, can be addicting.

Carefully read the patient information sheet that comes with the product. If you have any adverse side effects, contact your doctor immediately.

Be aware that your medications may need adjustment when you stop smoking.

If you have a contraindicated condition, such as pregnancy (nicotine in any form can harm the fetus), heart disease, allergies to drugs, very high blood pressure, stomach ulcers, overactive thyroid, diabetes, kidney or liver disease, you should know that both the SmokEnder program and the patch/gum work by reducing nicotine in the body. You may want to follow the regular SmokEnder program instead.

Both methods work to reduce the level of nicotine in your system, which prevents the physical craving and most of the withdrawal symptoms.

The patch or gum won't help you *stay* free of tobacco. It just weans you off nicotine so you can concentrate on disconnecting all the behavioral components of your habit: the psychological/emotional/habitual/oral/social/etc.

Don't allow yourself to believe that the patch/gum can take care of the problem alone. In fact, health agencies and patch makers agree that the patch/gum should be used *only* in conjunction with a comprehensive behavioral support program. That's what this book and program are all about.

If you are on the patch, for the purposes of this method consider this is the first day of the program.

Note to Cigar and Pipe Smokers and Smokeless Tobacco Users:

There are obvious differences between cigarette smoking and other tobacco uses. In any case, the following activities are essential in your effort to break free of your habit. Follow each step as closely as you can. Adapt where possible. There will be specific instructions along the way as necessary.

In all cases, patch/gum users and cigar/pipe/smokeless

users, use your good judgment and you'll do fine. This will work for you, too. *But you must work the program.*

Consider the importance of dealing with the psychological dependency, which in the final analysis is the one that causes smokers to resume smoking long after nicotine is out of their systems. How often I would quit for a week or two—the nicotine completely gone from my system—and the craving would become more and more intense, so I'd find an excuse to start smoking again. It was the psychological web that had me. It's easy to cut free, when you know how!

First, let's review what you've found out about smokers in general, and about yourself as a smoker. Check off those statements that express your feelings.

☐ You very likely have discovered that you really would like to quit smoking. You are probably disgusted with the habit for a lot more reasons than when you started reading this book. There's no question you'd exchange the habit for freedom from all the nuisance and problems. You can't seem to justify smoking to yourself any longer.

☐ You have sorted out the reasons you started to smoke as a youngster and found they had nothing to do with your current reasons for continuing to smoke—for instance, reverse peer pressure (interesting that it may have been peer pressure that got you smoking; now it's working to get you to quit!). And the consequent social unacceptability, so you're embarrassed to smoke in front of intelligent people . . . you hate feeling like a second-class citizen . . . huddled outside in the cold, rain and snow for a fix . . . and it's too much of a hassle to smoke anymore . . . and/or the disturbing feeling that you're harming your family and co-workers with your secondhand smoke . . .

☐ You accept the fact that nicotine is addictive—and you're very likely rather pleased to learn as a result that your willpower is not in question. You've learned that nicotine is generally out of your system within three or four days, and you will be prepared to deal with that as a transient problem. You know you won't "climb the walls."

☐ You've thought about the physical dangers of smoking (everything from fires to lung cancer) and you've realized how dependent you are upon your cigarettes, because you smoke in spite of your intelligence.

☐ Something new may be bothering you now: the horrible

awareness that if you become one of the unlucky ones, you will have done it to yourself—because there's no longer any question that many cancers, respiratory and heart problems are self-inflicted, by smoking.

☐ You are now cognizant of your responsibility to take charge of your own lifestyle and health—and to avoid harming your others with side-stream smoke from your burning tobacco.

☐ You've become aware of all the other habits that attached themselves to your smoking habit, like coffee, cola, alcohol, and you don't like having been shoved into doing things you can't easily control.

☐ You've also recognized how much of an automaton you've become by reaching for a cigarette whenever you get a signal or cue, such as the ringing of the telephone or clink of the coffee cup. Most likely you resent being outer-directed instead of inner-directed.

☐ You've learned about the power of the cigarette ads on your psyche and your consumer nerve. You'll soon be truly immune to the ads, but in the meantime you're defusing their power by satirizing them.

☐ The idea of quitting as tangible evidence of your self-mastery has great appeal. You're toying with the possibility that quitting smoking may also be an exhilarating experience.

☐ You now understand the relationship between smoking and weight gain and know that you don't necessarily gain weight because you quit—and you won't use that excuse as a cop-out for not quitting.

☐ You've learned that you're not alone. Hundreds of thousands of smokers have felt the way you do at this point. They couldn't imagine themselves not smoking. And they couldn't believe they could ever quit. But they did. And you can too.

☐ You've begun to imagine yourself as a non-smoker. You should now develop a mind-set in which smoking is an impediment to your desires.

☐ You have stopped telling yourself, "I enjoy smoking"; instead you acknowledge the fact that you're generally disgusted with the habit and wish you could quit. You know now that your "enjoyment" is really the relief of your self-induced discomfort because your body is crying out for a nicotine fix.

☐ You've begun to sell yourself on the idea of quitting as a positive experience—and to persuade yourself that you really *want* to quit.

☐ You've learned techniques for dealing with stress without using your cigarette as an amulet and cure-all.

☐ You've analyzed your own personal use of cigarettes and reasons for smoking, and you discovered it isn't the cigarette that gets things done or protects you. You've realized it's *you* and your own ability, personality, intelligence that are responsible for your success. You have begun to suspect you might even be more capable without the impediment of a cigarette to slow you down or drug your mind.

☐ You've learned that smoking doesn't make anything better. It doesn't make bad news better or fix broken objects, for instance.

☐ You understand now why smoking doesn't calm you down or steady your nerves. In fact, you realize that smoking, plus coffee, tea or cola, makes you more nervous and jittery.

☐ You've learned that those rationalizations we all use to protect the habit are downright silly. It would be difficult for you ever again to use one of those excuses without feeling foolish. And as an added support, you will laugh when you hear other smokers make the same statements and use the same phrases you used to.

☐ And most of all, you've learned that you must treat yourself with respect. You must convince yourself you're worth every effort. And in order to show that respect, you will reward yourself frequently, set worthy goals for your talents and ambitions, not allow yourself the childishness of self-pity or martyrdom and choose to live your life by your own command, instead of the cigarette's. You have decided that smoking will no longer dominate your existence. You want to be your own person.

If you're able to check off most of those statements as ones with which you agree, you're ready to quit. Jump right into the next stage. You should now make up your mind that you're going to stop once and for all. Remember, there is no perfect time to quit, either. If you wait until your life smooths out, you'll never quit.

Now look back at the list and study those items you DIDN'T check. Work at achieving the particular attitude that seems to have eluded you. Very often those unchecked items are the ones that block your best success.

First, before I get into specifics, let me lay down some general basic steps:

1. You might want to team up with a friend, but be very certain his or her interest in quitting is at a peak, or he'll pull you down. At the very least, he should read this book before doing it so you're both approaching it with a positive attitude. If you'd like to put a little group together write for a "Facilitator's Guide." See page 240 in "A Final Note from Jackie" in back of the book for information.

If you are a very private person, you might prefer to go it alone.

2. By now you have a little notebook with notes and lists from prior work. Carry it with you at all times; use it as you go along in the program. Refer to it or add data wherever you are.

In the following instructions, wherever a statement is in **BOLD CAPITALS,** write it in your notebook.

3. Choose a time and day of the week that will be a fixed "appointment" for the next five weeks. Allow about an hour a week to read the instructions and comply with them. It's important that you move from step to step a week at a time. Mark your calendar and honor the weekly date as if you have an appointment with a very important person. You do!

4. Set a date four weeks plus one day from the date you've set to start. For instance, let's say that your first "appointment" is Tuesday the eighth. The subsequent dates are the fifteenth, twenty-second, twenty-ninth and fifth. "Plus one day" means that you will be finished with smoking on the sixth. In the SmokEnders program, we call that your "Cut-Off" date. You'll never forget that date.

Once you've set the date, *write it in your workbook:* "**I will stop smoking on _____ (date)**" and circle it on all your calendars. It will be sacred. *NOTHING* should interfere with it. Don't consider changing it.

You might want to announce the date to all your friends and coworkers, but I suggest you work at this quietly and privately. What you don't need is outside pressure. In addition, I've learned that one of the serious obstacles to quitting is the malice of some smoking friends. If they hear that you're quitting, they become alarmed and, perhaps from subconscious motives, offer you cigarettes—blow smoke in your face—tease you for being "chicken" and afraid of cancer. (Your best weapon against their sabotage is understanding. They're afraid they'll be the last smoker in the office or car pool or bridge club.)

5. **Plan to do something very special** for yourself on your Cut-Off date. Please yourself. Don't think of your family or obligations just now. Begin thinking of things you'd enjoy and *write them in your workbook*.

6. During the time between now and your big date, begin to condition yourself physically and emotionally for the big event. In addition, physical activity helps detoxify you by moving the nicotine out of your system. It is a super weight control.

• Step up your circulation by **additional exercise.** Jumping jacks and jumping rope are the next best thing to cross-country skiing for maximum results. Start with a few, and build up as you get stronger. Join an aerobics group or a gym. Racquetball is an easy, fun game. I love it. Use a stair climber or a treadmill three to five times a week. At the very least, do the "Karma Stretches" every morning. (Refer to the Appendices.) Walking briskly is perhaps the best, because it's easy and convenient—all you need is some good walking shoes. Start with five minutes a day, maybe at lunch time—or any time it's convenient. Add a few minutes a day, and you'll soon be up to fifteen minutes and loving it. It feels *so good* to have your circulation going. And since that makes you breathe more often and more deeply, it's not only beneficial for healing your poor overworked lungs, but it acts to detoxify your body of nicotine and the thousands of toxic chemicals you've taken in from smoking. Another benefit of increasing your circulation: weight loss. It fires up your metabolism.

• **Begin drinking water regularly**—clear, cold water when you get up, before each meal (great weight control too. It sends a "full" signal, sooner) and several times during the day. Keep a distinctive glass on the sink to remind you. I keep a wine carafe filled with water on my desk now, because I enjoy it as some people enjoy having a Coke going all day long. Sometimes I put a slice of lemon or lime or mint leaves in it.

The water not only aids your circulation, which in turn adds oxygen to your blood, it also improves your bowel function and digestive system, helps flush your kidneys and, by cleansing the poisons out of your system more rapidly, makes you look and feel better! Now there's a miracle drug.

• **Avoid fatigue.** As you learned in Chapter 7, fatigue is another big cause of smoking. The cigarette people know that. Their ads told us to reach for a cigarette for "a lift." (They didn't tell us that one lift wouldn't be enough—because after a momentary lift we'd be more fatigued after each succeeding cigarette.)

Refer to "Instant Go" in the Appendices for healthy quick-energy ideas.

So, during the next four weeks, be sure to get plenty of rest and to eat frequent small, light, nourishing meals.

• **Try to avoid sugar and sugary foods,** which, for a variety of reasons, make you feel *hungry* and tired—both of which are powerful smoking "triggers." This is another important weight control.

• **Cut down on sodium**—not just the salt shaker, but high sodium foods, like smoked meats and fish, ham, processed foods, salted nuts, cheese, pickles, potato chips, pretzels with salt, soy sauce, etc. In my experience, salt has a greater effect on the body shortly after quitting than normally, so you may retain fluid and feel swollen and fat. Fluid retention also causes a variety of emotional reactions, such as tension, stress, temper, low moods, etc., similar to premenstrual tension. Naturally, it stands to reason that if your body is swollen with fluid, you're swollen all over—even your brain! And you're uncomfortable. Since one of the big reasons we smoke is to relieve physical and emotional discomfort, reducing sodium can make it easier for you to Cut-Off and stay off.

7. I don't believe it's necessary to live like a monk in order to quit smoking, or to refrain from alcohol or caffeine (coffee, cola, tea). It's a good idea, however to **reduce the quantity of caffeine and alcohol**—if you drink them regularly. Here's why:

Caffeine is a stimulant. It gives many people "coffee nerves." Most people smoke to relieve anxiety and tension. Less caffeine will make you calmer. One less reason to reach for a cigarette. Caffeine also dehydrates the body. When you're dehydrated, you look and feel rotten.

If you're concerned about weight, you should know that

caffeine is also an *appetite stimulant*! So much for all those diets that encouraged you to have all the coffee you wanted.

Incidentally, don't eliminate caffeine sharply. This is no time for additional withdrawal symptoms.

Alcohol is a depressant. Takes the edge off things, for a moment. But since nicotine is largely a stimulant, when you stop smoking, alcohol has a greater kick. There's no nicotine to counterbalance it. Also, alcohol tends to soften your resolve. "Ah, what's the difference? One little cigarette won't hurt, just this time." But most relapsed smokers know that it only took one little cigarette to get them right back on their two pack a day habit. So, if you feel obliged to drink (or *must* drink?), water it down, using more mixer than alcohol. If you're at a party, have the first drink watered down, then order juice with a straw or swizzle stick, or Perrier and lime, or so on. Another weight control, too.

A final argument to help you decide to reduce the coffee, cola, tea and booze for now: they are all strong smoking "triggers."

8. Begin to **develop strong personal, selfish, ego reasons** for wanting to quit. Reasons that will offer you benefits beyond self-preservation and obligation. One of my most powerful reasons (not the most powerful—that was extremely personal) was that I didn't want to become a little-old-lady smoker. I hate the look of it. So you see, "good" reasons may not have anything to do with your health. Motivation is the key to your success. Find reasons that are meaningful to you. Not *intellectual* reasons. Not *self-righteous* reasons. Gut reasons. Ego reasons. Vanity reasons.

For some good ideas, go back to Chapter 13. All are great reasons. If any strikes a nerve, make it yours.

Don't get stuck in the trap of thinking a reason must be profound, for example: "to avoid lung cancer." Obviously for most smokers that's been one of the primary reasons for wanting to quit—but you, and they, are still smoking. So that's not a good reason to quit; it's a swell reason to enjoy *not* smoking after you quit!

In your notebook on the top of a fresh page, write **REASONS TO QUIT SMOKING.** Begin to list every reason that comes to mind. The smallest, silliest reason may be the most powerful motivator for you. Add to this list whenever another reason hits you. For example, the next time you get out of breath running up the stairs, say, "I'll be glad when I don't smoke so I have better stamina." Or the next time you have to go outside to smoke because your smoking isn't welcome in the home you're visiting, say, "I hate having to do this. I really want to quit so I don't have to get a fix."

9. Begin to **plan lovely non-smoking, non-food rewards** for yourself. Not for your spouse or kids or parents. For YOU. You must repattern your reward reflex, so when you stop smoking, you don't reach for a cigarette when you really want to do something nice for yourself.

You see, one of the big reasons we smoke is to give ourselves a treat: a reward for a job done; for a tiring phone call; for a heavy feeling of self-pity . . . whatever. **Begin a list of rewards** and treats to which you can refer during this quitting process, and after you quit, when you feel an impulse to smoke.

About five pages after the REASONS page, head another page with **REWARDS.** Every time you think "I wish I could . . ." write it on your Rewards list. For instance, "Could find time to read a new book; play with the kids; buy a new record; go fishing; call a friend; do my knitting; travel around the world; etc." It doesn't have to cost anything to be a good reward, but you will save a lot of money when you stop smoking, and we urge you to spend it on yourself—frivolously. After all, you used to burn it up—now you can use it for anything you'd like and not feel guilty spending it.

Have plenty of quick and easy Rewards—things that take less than five minutes, because the impulse to smoke only lasts three or four minutes, and if you distract yourself—it passes!

10. **BEGIN A GRATITUDE LIST.** To defeat self-pity, a powerful negative emotion to which most of us succumb when we quit without proper preparation, it's necessary to focus on the good in our lives. You have so much to live for—and so much to look forward to—but you must examine your life from time to time to remind yourself of all you have. Even if the chips are down, you have a lot. Everyone does. Here is the exercise to bring your gratitude level up, and to thwart self-pity.

If you haven't yet started a list of "assets" start one now. Title the page ASSETS—THINGS I VALUE IN MY LIFE. Later, when you go through your notebook to do the work of the day, make a list of all those things that are meaningful to you. Start with your family, your dog, good job, have a good friend, etc., what you own, (like "Great House," "Nice Car," etc.), and then the personal qualities of which you're proud: great complexion, fine head of hair, nice build, terrific eyes, teeth, smile . . . Then your talents: nice personality, a musical aptitude, good at sports, good sense of humor. And then your health . . . the fact that you're not in the hospital . . .

As you think of things for which to be grateful, write them in your book. Then, when you hear yourself saying, "Poor me, I can't have a cigarette," and you have a childish tantrum, you can laugh at yourself and remember all the wonderful things you have and are. It's pretty hard to feel sorry for yourself when you are grateful.

11. Although you will find *weight controls* built into this program, if you're terribly concerned about gaining weight, put yourself on a simple, efficient weight-loss program for a few weeks before you start this program. Then if you should happen to gain, it won't become an excuse to start smoking again. Still, if you do gain weight, remember that quitting is far more important, from a health point of view: You would have to gain between 75 and 125 extra pounds to do the damage to your heart and body that smoking a pack a day does.

I didn't gain weight when I quit—but then I had been aware that I gained whenever I went cold-turkey in the past, so I built a lot of tricks into this program to keep me from having that excuse to start smoking again. Do everything you're asked to do, and the chances are good you won't gain. You see, if you quit smoking without feeling deprived, you won't substitute food to try to make up for the loss. I truly believe it's far better to concentrate on quitting and then on losing weight. One thing at a time, or the mind and body get cranky and stubborn. And your newfound sense of self-mastery gives you a wonderful feeling that "If I can quit smoking I can do anything!" So you can go on to lose weight or write that book or go back for your degree.

My mail is full of wonderful letters from people who write that SmokEnders and/or this book—was the best thing they ever did for themselves because it got them started moving in a forward direction in their lives: better jobs, better relationships, able to take more risks, got degrees, changed careers, started body building and other self-improvement activities . . . and so on. You can use quitting as a catalyst, too. If you've always wanted to lose weight, do it after you stop smoking. (Interestingly, many SmokEnders had weight problems before they quit smoking, and some others gained as a result of quitting; so many of them asked me to write a program like SmokEnders for weight control. I hope to have DietEnders published soon. If you want to be informed when it's available, see page 240.)

12. From now on, look at smokers as if you've never seen anyone smoke before. Pretend you just landed from another planet. After a while, you'll see that smoking looks kind of silly . . . that most people don't look like Mr. Macho, or Ms. Glamour. Most don't look cool and sophisticated. Those that do would look that way without a cigarette. Most smokers look pale and pasty. Also, nicotine is like a leather tanning agent. It toughens the skin and wrinkles it prematurely. Some are squinty-eyed because the smoke is drifting into their eyes. Then there are those with stained teeth, and when you stop smoking, you'll get a whiff of foul smoker's breath. (You may not be sensitive to it now because when you smoke your olfactory nerve—your sense of smell—is sort of paralyzed.)

After you watch enough smokers, begin to pity them. That's preparation for after you quit. I used to envy smokers every time I was off cigarettes. I thought, how lucky they were that they could smoke freely, without having to quit . . . like me. When I finally saw smoking through different eyes, I didn't envy smokers any more. And when I finally stopped smoking, I pitied them. If they only knew how nice it felt to be free of cigarettes.

Pity smokers. After you quit, it will fall into place. And incidentally, it will keep you from becoming an obnoxious "reformed" smoker.

13. **Visualize yourself as a non-smoker.** There was a time you didn't smoke. It was the real you. From now on, keep

thinking how nice it will be when you're not bothered with the nuisance or worry about smoking. See yourself fresh and clean and full of new energy. You'll be surprised at how much more stamina and vitality you have when you stop. Because you probably started smoking in your teens, YOU DON'T KNOW WHAT IT'S LIKE TO BE AN ADULT NON-SMOKER. And that's the good news: *your body will restore itself very quickly* (unless you have cancer or emphysema, which is irreversible). For instance, if you have a cough or hack, it will most likely disappear within the first week of not smoking! Color will return to your cheeks. Your eyes will look whiter and brighter. People will comment on how well you look. It's amazing.

The important attitude at this juncture is to view quitting as an addition to your personality and well-being rather than something you have given up. Then, if the thought of a cigarette comes to mind after you quit, you will have a ready mind-set: "Not me—*I DON'T SMOKE ANYMORE! I ENJOY MY FREEDOM FROM SMOKING.*"

Quitting Smoking Is Not a Single Act—It Is a Process

The following detoxification and behavior modification techniques are broken down into four stages, to be completed one week apart. This gives your *mind* time to unlearn your old habit and learn your new non-smoking habit—and your *body* time to detoxify from the nicotine slowly and gently.

Be kind to your mind and body and work at this as *the most important activity in your life for the next several weeks*. It surely is worth it. You surely are worth it.

I'd like you to assess your state of mind, now, and to make a commitment to yourself and to me. Check off the following if you agree:

☐ Quitting smoking is the most important thing in my life for the next four weeks.
☐ I believe that I have a sincere personal desire to quit.
☐ I will be honest with myself throughout this process.
☐ I will keep an open mind—I won't let skepticism block my success.

☐ I will persevere, no matter what, because I'm determined to break free.
☐ I will do exactly what I'm told to do. Not more. Not less.

Sometimes people think that if they do more—or are hard on themselves—they'll get better results and some people feel they "understand" the concept and so skip it. Remember, this is easy, if you follow the program. It doesn't have to hurt to work! Agreed? Okay. Then Ready, Set, GO!

WEEK ONE

1. You must continue to smoke until the day after your fifth session, but this week **change your brand** to any other brand(s) with which you're comfortable. Stay within the *nicotine* range of your current brand but not more than 1.0 mg. Refer to the Federal Trade Commission chart in the back of the book. (If you are reading this after 1995, I suggest you call or write the FTC in Washington, D.C., for an updated version. The Public Reference Branch of the FTC, Sixth Street and Pennsylvania Avenue, N.W., Washington, DC, 20580, (202) 326-2000 or (202) 326-2222. Or ask your librarian. Or read the nicotine rating in the cigarette ads.)

Buy several packs. A variety of brands or all the same. Enough for the week, but don't buy by the carton anymore.

Don't try to cut down. If you want to smoke, light up.

2. Now the "magic" starts:

Remove Pack Strap #1 from the chart section in the back of the book. Find a golf or bridge pencil or **make a "short" pencil** by cutting a regular pencil in half—about the length of a cigarette.

Wrap the chart around the pack of cigarettes you're now smoking. Cover just the sides of the pack, not the top, so you can easily obtain a cigarette. Secure it with a rubber band. (Covering the pack eliminates one big cause of reaching for a cigarette without thinking: the familiar artwork on the pack is a major trigger!)

Drop the pencil in the pack.

Each time you take a cigarette, the pencil will pop out to remind you to **make a "hash mark" (a slash) under the hour of the day you are lighting up.** After you mark the chart, light up. That way you won't forget to do it. It's very important that you record each cigarette as you have it. (Don't try to remember. It doesn't work.) When you finish a pack, slide the Pack Strap off and slide it on a new pack.

This exercise will help you identify your smoking patterns, so please smoke all you want. It doesn't do to deny yourself.

At the end of your week, total across and down for the week. Don't discard the Pack Strap.

Note: If you're using the Patch or Nicorette, don't smoke. Just mark the times you have an *impulse* to smoke.

3. **Mark a T for Taste** instead of a hash-mark any time a cigarette tastes delicious. Mark it only *after* you light up and assess the taste. You'll be surprised at the results.

4. At the end of each meal—whatever you consider the last gulp or bite—even if it's just a cup of coffee, look at your watch and determine the time. **Delay smoking for just fifteen minutes.** This is surprisingly easy because you can have as many as you want when the time is up.

This is the beginning of putting space between a condition (the end of the meal) and your usual response (lighting up). You'll be very proud to have some control of cigarettes, even in one short week.

5. Instead of sitting at the table thinking of a cigarette (or ogling dessert!) after every meal brush your teeth with a good, fresh toothpaste, then rinse with a pungent mouthwash, undiluted. Not too sweet or medicinal. It's helpful to floss too, to get all the food particles out. They can trigger a desire for a cigarette too. Prepare a portable Oral Gratification Kit: carry a portable toothbrush, small tube of toothpaste and small bottle of mouthwash in a little plastic case or Ziplock.

This is also a terrific distracting technique. You will have used up fifteen minutes without counting the seconds until you can have a cigarette—and you have a wonderful, clean mouth taste. Now you can smoke all you like, but that clean mouth isn't conducive to smoking, so you might go well past fifteen minutes now and then. Your old habit is starting to disintegrate already!

And you've taken a good step toward *controlling your weight,* because you're attending to your mouth. The need for oral gratification is very strong when you quit because your mouth is used to having something put in it every few minutes all day long. For instance, if you put each cigarette to your mouth about ten times, and you smoke a pack a day, you touch your mouth about 200 times a day—73,000 a year—1,400,000 in twenty years! No wonder people stuff their mouths with food, pencils, eyeglasses, gum, anything, when they quit cold-turkey!

Plan to do your oral hygiene routine after each meal—no matter what. Even if you're at a restaurant or the office.

Also buy a little portable breath spray for emergencies.

But remember, the more you brush, rinse and floss, the more satisfied your mouth will be when you stop smoking—and the more comfortable you'll be as a non-smoker.

Don't cut any corners. The more you put into this the better your result. And you deserve to be free.

6. Because you're not smoking immediately after your meal, you might need Tums for a while because your digestive system is caught by surprise without nicotine to shock it into motion. Your body will soon take over its natural housekeeping and the acidity will disappear. In fact, many people with peptic ulcers are delighted to find the ulcers disappear when they quit smoking.

Similarly, you might need a laxative for a while, for the same reason. No nicotine shock. Happily, your system responds positively within a week or so.

So plan to **carry Tums or other antacid tablets.** And eat bran or drink prune juice each morning.

Don't allow yourself to become uncomfortable in any way. Remember, one of the reasons we smoke is to relieve discomfort. *Any* discomfort.

7. Each night before falling asleep, review your notebook. Write more good reasons for wanting to quit smoking, more ideas for rewards. Then **write your thoughts as in a journal.** State your feelings to yourself. This book is very personal. Nobody should ever look at it, so you can express your deepest feelings. Are you fearful of quitting? Hopeful? Ambivalent? What are your hopes? Your worries? What are you angry about? What do you want? Open up your heart. Be honest with yourself. This is very important to your "cure."

And before falling asleep, advertise to yourself:

> I really want to quit smoking—
> I *will* stop smoking—
> and I'm looking forward to being free.

Note: Resist reading next week's instructions until this time next week.

WEEK TWO

You've come a long way, baby! Believe it or not, you've made wonderful progress already. Here's what you've done:

- You put space between conditions and responses by delaying smoking for fifteen minutes after meals. Now you have some hope that you can control your smoking habit. Your feeling of hopelessness and helplessness is lifting. That's important because if you believe you will fail, you will; if you believe you can succeed, you will.
- You have begun to retrain your mouth by brushing and flossing after each meal. That clean mouth taste is hard to beat—it sort of makes smoking the next cigarette, pipe or cigar less appealing. This mouth satisfaction process will go a long way toward your weight control too.
- You probably cut down on your cigarette consumption because of the chart, which made you aware of each cigarette. As a result, you have begun gently to reduce the amount of nicotine in your system. That's why it's important that you continue to smoke and don't cut down too sharply.
- You changed your brand—so your "old buddy" brand has lost its power over you.
- Count the number of T's on your Pack Strap. Are you surprised how few cigarettes tasted good? Though the cigarette ads tell us we smoke for taste—the reality is we smoke because we're addicted to the nicotine in the tobacco.

You're doing fine. The important thing this week is for you to persevere. Don't waver—and don't anticipate. Do everything in these instructions—nothing more, nothing less. In just a few weeks you'll be free of cigarettes and can return to your old ways—without smoking.

1. In Chapter 4 you were asked to list the ways you "use" smoking. Now on that page, write in yourself notebook, **"Why I smoke—what I like about it."** Think of all the reasons you smoke and write them down.

2. On another page write, **"What I've gotten from smoking** (the price I'm paying for smoking)." Here are a few starter ideas: a hacking cough; more short-winded so I don't do sports anymore; my clothes smell; I worry about my breath and musty body odor; worry about my health; fear of cancer; guilty feelings about setting a bad example; my house has a

stale smell; could have a nice car or vacation for the money I spend on cigarettes, etc. As you think of other high costs of feeling lousy, write them down.

3. **Calculate the cost of smoking.** Use the worksheet in the back of the book to figure the amount of money you've spent on smoking so far, and then the amount you *will* spend if you continue to smoke. I caution you: it's a shocking experience. (Patch and gum users—calculate what you will save because you have quit.)

Even now, before state and the federal governments start loading on taxes to help with the cost of health care, cigarettes—at $2.00 to $2.50 a pack in U.S. and U.K. (six dollars in Canada)—are no longer just an incidental expense. For instance, if you smoke the average one and a half packs a day, at two dollars per pack, you spend $90 a month on cigarettes. If there are two smokers in your family, that's $180 a month! And $2,160 a year! (Not counting the costs of maintaining the smoking habit.)

My son, Peter, a financial planner now working toward his MBA at Yale, became interested in the hard numbers relative to the cost of smoking. He got to thinking about all that money to be saved and created some spreadsheets showing interest compounded at various interest rates. He wrote to me explaining his assumptions, briefly as follows: "If an individual starts smoking at age twenty-five [he doesn't know that most people start before they're eighteen], and continues until retirement at age sixty-five, that's forty years." In this example he assumes 2½ packs for 40 years at $4 average per pack, at 7% average annual interest. "That comes to over **three-quarters of a million dollars.** Perhaps I am thinking like a broke grad student, but that's a heap of cash in my opinion." He adds, "If someone who is looking for the 'trick' says, 'Well, after inflation, how much is that really going to be worth in forty years?' I respond, 'You're right, it won't feel like as much then as now. Let's say inflation cuts that in half. It will feel like somewhere between $350,000 and $400,000 today. Which would you rather have in forty years—$350,000 more or $350,000 less?'

"If the average two-pack-a-day smoker smoked $3.00 of cigarettes, quit and handed the same money over to a financial planner who was moderately competent, the chances are very good that there would be enough money saved and compounded over twenty years to fund their child's Ivy League education, or to buy that cabin in the mountains, or to substantially increase their retirement fund.

"Compounding interest is like a fungus. It just grows on itself and multiplies without interference. The trick is for smokers to routinely put the money away—every week, if possible, or certainly every month. And the sooner the better, because time is the element that makes compounding magic."

For now, decide to do something *frivolous* with the money you'll have saved in three months after you quit. A wonderful, personal REWARD. Then continue to save your cigarette money faithfully. Perhaps at the end of one year celebrate by taking a very special trip with that $1,400 more or less. Look at it this way: You'd find the money for tobacco; you smoke for a reward; cigarette smoking is a frivolous way to burn up money; reward yourself in a new way with that money.

Think of it as paying dues in a different club. You quit the cigarette club and have joined a new club that is dedicated to serving *you* in clean, healthful, satisfying ways instead of unnecessary sickness, dirtiness and possibly premature death.

(Yes, you must become a bit of self-indulgent during this phase. You are asked to be nice to yourself in new ways, to consider your needs, and to become more assertive. We often use smoking as a smoke screen to obscure our feelings.)

4. In observing smokers last week, did you see many that looked like the ads: Mr. Macho, Ms. Clean and Healthy and Sexy? Probably not. Most smokers look pale, tense, tired. Some smell pretty bad. (But you might not know that until you stop smoking, because your sense of smell is dulled by smoking.) Can you let go of the old image of smoking as glamorous and grown-up? Begin to see it as the weird thing it is: inhaling gases and particulate matter from burning leaves held together by a piece of chemically treated paper. When you let go of the old image, you'll watch people smoke and see it as the "funny" thing it is. And you'll begin to pity them.

5. **On last week's Pack Strap add the columns down and across.** Total the amount smoked, or the number of impulses, if you're on the patch or gum, for the week.

Start a new page in your notebook, head it "Amount Smoked Per Week," write Week 1, 2, 3, 4, on the left side of the page. Each week, write the total number smoked as recorded on your Pack Strap.

Now circle **the three highest numbers** in the last column. These are your peak stress periods. Probably it will be something like ten to eleven in the morning, and three to four in the afternoon, and eight to nine at night. These are the most common times for most people—smokers or not. And there's a reason: fatigue causes most mid-morning and mid-afternoon slumps. Boredom/TV watching causes the evening peak period. You may have stress periods other than those I mentioned, but you must determine the cause, and act to do what is needed, instead of using a cigarette.

Study your weekend patterns too. Do you smoke more—or less on weekends? What does that tell you?

Start a new page, head it "Stress Periods." Write the hours of the peak periods and the cause as you determine it, like this:

1. 4:00 P.M.   kids fussy time, I'm fatigued
2. 11:00 A.M.   tired, hungry
3. 9–9:30 P.M. bored, TV watching

Notice that the hours are not in chronological order. They are in order of the highest of the three peak times to the lowest.

For help with your stress periods, refer to "Tools to Cope" in back of the book. If possible, make a copy and carry it with you so you can refer to it when you identify a "stressor."

This is the beginning of learning how to cope without cigarettes—stress management.

6. **This second week, observe self-pity in others and in yourself.** It's a very destructive, negative emotion, and very childish. It's important that you don't allow self-pity to control you during this quitting phase. President Eisenhower

said when he quit smoking, "If you don't feel sorry for yourself, it isn't nearly as hard to quit."

It really is the attitude posture you take regarding quitting. Understanding this concept was a turning point for me.

You aren't "giving up" something of value. You're really gaining many good things by quitting, not least of which is self-mastery. It is probably the most gratifying feeling in the world—because when you quit smoking, you will know that *you did it by yourself*. No one else can do it for you. Even after all the years since I quit smoking, I rank quitting as one of the most important things I've done in my life. And thousands of people write to say thanks for "changing my life for the better and *incidentally* for helping me quit smoking."

Here's how to deal with self-pity when you see it:

• Think of all the good things in your life. It's hard to feel sorry for yourself when you're grateful. Refer to your list of "Assets" and "Accomplishments."

• Laugh at it. It's so childish. It's hard to feel sorry for yourself when you're laughing.

Here are your instructions for the week:

1. **Prepare Pack Strap #2.** Smoke as much as you like. This time, in addition to recording all your cigarettes, **mark an A for every alcoholic drink** (beer, wine and hard liquor) and a **C for any caffeine** intake. Remember, caffeine is coffee, regular tea and cola. Don't bother marking decaffeinated or herbal beverages.

Be certain to mark *all* cigarettes *before* you light up. Don't try to recall any cigarettes "later" or to estimate at the end of the day. You're only fooling yourself that way.

2. **Change your brand to one you dislike,** but no higher than 0.8 mg, as shown on the FTC chart in the back of the book. For instance, if you're a menthol smoker, switch to a non-menthol, or vice-versa; go from filter to non-filter. Or just switch to brands you always said you disliked. (Curiously, you're likely to find that they're really okay after you smoke a pack or two. After all, they please a lot of other people. So much for taste and brand loyalty.) If you're on a low nicotine brand, don't switch to any higher.

3. If you aren't smoking right now, light one up. Observe yourself smoking. With which hand do you smoke? In what side of your mouth do you put the cigarette?

If you always smoke with the cigarette in your right hand, change to your left. (This is fun when you try to drink coffee backward too!) Also put your cigarette into the opposite side of your mouth. From now on, smoking isn't going to be automatic. Awareness is an important psychological technique. It will help you immensely. **So change hand and side of mouth.**

4. Keep your cigarettes in a different pocket or drawer. Just **change the location** so its unfamiliar. Don't make it inconvenient. If they're hard to get, you will lose patience and it won't work.

5. **Pack away all your smoking accessories:** lighters, cases, whatever. Save them because someday they'll be relics of a bygone age. Cigarette smoking is becoming as unfashionable as chewing tobacco. Maybe soon there will be only closet smokers. Studies show that less people in the upper socio-economic strata smoke cigarettes now; the revolution is happening fast. Another good reason to quit smoking.

6. **Delay smoking for one-half hour** after each meal, after awakening in the morning, and before going to sleep at night.

If you are a pre-breakfast smoker, a good trick is to put a thermos of undiluted lemon juice on your night table. One swig of that in the morning will get you started—better than the jolt you get from nicotine.

Another helpful trick: brush your teeth AFTER your last cigarette of the night. Then your mouth won't taste like the bottom of a bird cage when you wake up and you won't need a cigarette to relieve that discomfort. Quickly, upon awakening, brush your teeth vigorously and rinse with a strong mouthwash.

To help you get past the bedtime cigarette ritual, try repatterning to have a warm, soothing bath just before bed. Or do something pleasant—a hobby, read your Reasons List, meditate, do the Relaxation Ritual—*after* you've had your last cigarette. *BUT, whenever you have your last cigarette, you must wait one-half hour before getting into bed or turning off the light*.

Watch for self-pity here. Laugh at it. When you have

overtaken these two well ingrained smoking rituals—morning and bedtime—you will be well on your way to winning this personal war.

7. **Begin drinking water**—at least four glasses a day. Start with just four ounces before each meal and any time you might reach for coffee or a cola drink. Your body is calling for water. Thirst is its signal. And the more water you drink, the more poisons are flushed out of your body. Another detoxification aid.

In addition to the above suggestions, remember to:

Reach for fructose or orange juice if you need a lift; every night read your Reasons for wanting to be free of cigarettes; get as much physical activity as you can—walk briskly at least fifteen minutes a day; get enough sleep; satisfy your mouth's needs by brushing your teeth and rinsing after every eating incident; observe smokers.

You're in training for your own personal Olympic challenge. You can do it, and you will. Don't let anything get in your way. Say to yourself over and over, "Quitting smoking is the best thing I can do for myself. I really want to quit so I'll do everything I'm supposed to do, without excuse."

Recite frequently:

> I will stop smoking
> I will look better
> I will feel better
> I will be FREE!

WEEK THREE

Review your Pack Strap. Add columns across and down. *Write the total smoked (or impulses if you're on the patch or gum) for the week in your notebook next to last week's.*

Compare it with prior week's totals. Did you smoke fewer cigarettes this week than last? Than the first week? If you have been hash-marking each cigarette before you light up, I know you have cut down, because awareness eliminates at least 20% of those we light up—without thinking. Then there's another 15% to 20% that, when you stop to think about it (because you have to make a hash mark), you don't really want one, after all—you figured out that you want/need something else. Perhaps you have quite naturally begun to *decode your cravings* by asking yourself, "What do I really want?" "What am I feeling?" "What would make me feel better right now?" To help you with this important technique, you'll find a list in the back of the book called "Tools to Cope": Decode. Distract. Repattern.

I suggest you use it to take positive action instead of taking a cigarette—and then, to prevent a lifetime occurrence of the situation—to repattern.

Back to the total smoked this week. Was the cut-down natural or was it self-imposed restraint? (What I call the "goody-goody" approach.) Please be certain that you smoke as many as you like, and don't restrain yourself if you want one—except during delay times—because, although you will stop smoking, you may not have the positive feeling that comes with quitting this way. If you feel you've denied yourself, your chance of starting to smoke again is stronger.

Now *circle the three highest numbers in the last column.* These are your peak Stress Periods. *Write the hours and possible causes in your notebook under last week's report of stress periods.*

Are your peak periods more clearly defined this week? How do your weekends fare? If you smoke more (or have more impulses) on weekends than during the week, you might think about repatterning your weekends. Something about it must either produce anxiety, too much socializing or, perhaps, boredom.

On the other hand, if you smoke less on weekends, it may be because you don't want to smoke as much in front of your family or in the house because of secondhand smoke, or because you smoke more at work. Is there something about your work that causes you to smoke more? Change whatever you can. Soon, however, if you live and work in the United States, it will be changed for you, as far as smoking at work is concerned. The government, through OSHA, is acting to restrict smoking in ALL workplaces in the U.S. Other countries have already done so, or will surely follow suit after the U.S. does. Studies show smoking increases down time and reduces productivity, so in the name of competition, if not citizen health, smoking will be banned in most of the developed countries within several years.

During delay times, have you mastered the distraction technique? This, too, is a clue to your commitment to quitting. If you sit and suffer the delay times, you are allowing yourself to suffer purposely. You are sabotaging yourself. Self-pity surely comes into play. If you get up from the table and brush your teeth—vigorously and lovingly—and then get busy doing something interesting to reward yourself, the time passes quickly. You will get a super result. Here, again, it's important for you to use "Tools to Cope" and your "Rewards" list to find positive solutions.

How many times did you go past the half-hour delay without realizing it? Great! It will happen more often this week, as you break more and more habit connectors.

Count the number of C's on Pack Strap #2. If you find more than three a day, you'll be pleased to watch the number diminish as you go along. As you cut out cigarettes, you automatically cut down on coffee and cola. Smokers use coffee to try to make the cigarettes taste better, and use cigarettes to try to make the coffee taste better! Also, when you quit smoking, you won't need a pick-up after a cigarette. So when you quit smoking, you break the caffeine habit or at least cut down on a heavy one. A nice bonus.

Count the number of A's. If you have alcohol every day, it might be a clue to another excess in your life. Most people have a drink or two a couple of times a week. Not every day. It's a good idea to water down your drinks while you're quitting smoking . . . or do without alcohol altogether for now. I remember I almost relapsed shortly after I quit because we were out celebrating my successful quitting— and I had two drinks. It packed a greater wallop without nicotine in my system . . . and I felt so relaxed and happy, I thought, "One won't hurt!" Fortunately, my husband didn't let me fall into that trap, and I survived as a non-smoker!

Did you smoke less during your peak periods this week because you took orange juice or fructose when you needed a lift? Did you repattern your routine so you had a good breakfast; got to bed on time; broke the bedtime cigarette ritual and the morning "kicker" cigarette? Did you identify any other causes of peak periods—and did you create a remedy?

Congratulations. You're doing fine. You're on your way to becoming a non-smoker—soon! PERSIST. This is the most important activity in your life—for just a few more weeks.

Here are your instructions for the week:

1. **Prepare Pack Strap #3.** Smoke as much as you like, but record all your cigarettes, plus all A's and C's. Mark it *before* you light up. Don't estimate at the end of the day. It doesn't work!

2. **Change your brand** to any that has .5 milligrams of nicotine or less. Forget about tar content now. Although it's the "tar" that's linked to cancer, you won't be smoking many more; it's the nicotine content that is important now. Nicotine is the addictive element. Buy enough for the week so you don't run out and have to make do with a brand that's not recommended. The FTC chart in the back of the book reflects nicotine ratings as of 1994. If you are reading this book more than two years past that date, I suggest you write to the Federal Trade Commission in Washington, D.C., and request a current rating sheet. Or ask your librarian. Better yet, read the cigarette ads. Cigarette companies are required by law to publish the tar and nicotine level in the ad. And we now know there are indications that the cigarette companies manipulate the amount of nicotine—to keep you hooked, although the cigarette companies still deny it.

3. **Delay smoking for three-quarters of an hour** after ALL food and beverages except the following: water, raw fruits and vegetables, milk, boullion and juice. None are "trig-

gers''; all are healthful and non-fattening and they all combat fatigue.

That means no more coffee *and* cigarette, or alcohol *and* cigarette. You may have either but not both together, and I'd prefer that you chose the cigarette! One more cigarette won't make much difference, but each dose of caffeine and alcohol you eliminate makes it much easier for you to succeed at gaining control of your smoking and your life!

4. **Delay smoking for three-quarters of an hour** before bedtime. A good time for a relaxation reward.

5. **No smoking BEFORE breakfast.** Your first cigarette will be three-quarters of an hour after breakfast. It helps if you brush your teeth before going to sleep at night—so you don't have a bad taste in your mouth in the morning, which is a trigger to smoke: to relieve another discomfort. Don't forget to keep a carafe of lemon and water on your night table if you're an early morning smoker.

Note regarding delay times: If you allow yourself to think of wanting a cigarette during the delay times, it is an indication of your willingness to indulge in self-pity—or a desire to suffer. Don't let the thought of a cigarette enter your mind. How? Distract yourself. Review "Tools to Cope" if necessary. Plan things to do that occupy your mind pleasantly ahead of time. Another reason to have a good list of rewards ready.

6. **No smoking during the night**—after going to bed. If you wake up, imagine a "No Smoking" sign in the bedroom; keep a thermos of warm milk on the night table, or take fructose. If you need more armament, imagine that you have set your house on fire. Thirty percent of all house fires in the United States are caused by cigarette smoking!

7. **Continue with oral gratification** after each meal and before bed, and use a breath spray after all snacks.

8. **Continue adding to your lists of Reasons and Rewards.** You will want to have good lists handy for future reinforcement purposes, too. Read your list of reasons. **Memorize the five most important reasons.** Begin to reward yourself in small ways. Take five minutes to call a good friend; buy yourself a flower; make an appointment to get a great new haircut; buy a new magazine; order tickets for a good play or concert; take a snooze; or a soothing bubble bath. Read

some trash and don't feel guilty! Be creative. Good rewards don't require lots of time or money.

9. **Firm up your plans for Cut-Off Day.** Take the day off if you can, unless you like the routine of work. In that case plan to do something wonderful to celebrate after work. You won't be climbing the walls, because the amount of nicotine remaining in your system will be insignificant. It will truly be a happy and exciting moment in your life.

10. **Continue to observe smokers,** and listen to their rationalizations. You will smile at the excuses they make to protect their smoking habit—and their egos. You know better now.

Remind yourself that you really WANT to quit smoking now, although it's not unusual for you to feel a bit ambivalent—a bit hopeful that you'll quit; yet a bit fearful that you will. Separating from a "beloved old buddy" can be viewed as unpleasant. But this is a buddy who, sooner or later, will betray you. Let go of it before it lets you have the worst of its favors!

Think instead of how fresh and clean and energetic and guilt-free you'll feel when you quit. Because I assure you, that's the payoff. It's wonderful not to smoke!

Frequently during the day and especially before falling asleep each night, reaffirm your commitment to yourself:

> I will stop smoking
> I will look better
> I will feel better
> and I will be FREE.

WEEK FOUR

How are you feeling this week? Your body may have begun to respond to the changes you're making. When it happened to me, I realized it was a sign that my body was recovering from all the years I'd "insulted" it with a powerful poison (nicotine), plus hundreds of chemicals used in creating a smokable cigarette, and particulate matter that came with the smoke. So instead of calling the physical reactions withdrawal pains, I called them "Symptoms of Recovery." I was so happy my body was able to recover from so many years of smoking.

You may not have any "symptoms of recovery" or you may have several. You may not have any until after you cut off, or you may have some now because you've substantially reduced the amount of nicotine in your bloodstream; also, you've likely cut down on caffeine which also plays havoc with your physical being.

If you're having any unusual physical reactions, like increased thirst, check the "Symptoms of Recovery" list in the back of the book. But the main piece of information is *Forewarned is Forearmed*: don't panic. Any unusual physical reaction will pass. If you're concerned or if it is not on the list, check with your doctor.

Even if you do nothing, your body will rebuild and restore itself to its normal healthy method of keeping you functioning—as if you had never smoked! Thank the good Lord your body is so forgiving.

A few of the more common "Symptoms of Recovery" of which you should be aware are: sudden drowsiness, muddleheadedness and bleeding gums. These are so common I feel it's necessary to mention them so you take it in stride.

1. Of greatest importance is sudden drowsiness if you drive a car or truck, or work at machinery. We recommend you carry a caffeine-based lozenge like Enerjets or No Doz. They work quickly, are always available, and although they contain caffeine, they aren't a trigger, as a cup of coffee would be. They are available at some drugstores and truck stops.

2. If your gums bleed, buy some Amosan at the drugstore.

If necessary, see your dentist for a deep scaling. Your gums are returning to normal too, and are sloughing off the hard casing they developed to protect tender tissue from the heat and toxins of smoking. If your dentist would like more information about this as yet unpublished information about bleeding gums, you may want to show him the "Bleeding Gums" letter from my husband, Jon Rogers, DDS. It's in the back of the book.

3. **For now, blame anything bad on cigarettes, anything good on quitting.** Your energy and vitality will soon improve, which is great. Your taste buds, too, for which I offer a caution: since food will taste so much better to you, you might not realize how much more you're eating. So choose carefully and eat wisely, and if you're concerned about weight gain, increase protein and eliminate simple carbohydrates (sugar and sugary foods).

If you are presently on any medication, don't change the dosage until after Cut-Off. This is no time to load yourself with additional physical or emotional strain.

Review your Pack Strap. Turn to the page on which you wrote the total number of cigarettes you smoked in the prior weeks and your earlier Stress Periods: Write this week's total smoked. Compare it with the past numbers. Can you see a reduction in quantity? That's wonderful as long as you aren't restraining yourself when you want a cigarette. This isn't a matter of tapering off, which doesn't work. I used to try that. I'd pledge to smoke only 39 one day, then 38 the next and so on, hoping to eliminate the whole habit when I got to zero. Problem was, when I got down to about eight a day, I couldn't give any more up. Each one was the MOST IMPORTANT. I really suffered, and in suffering, I needed more cigarettes.

You understand all that now, don't you? So don't try to taper off. This program says "smoke as many as you like" so you won't suffer. You will reduce the amount you smoke quite naturally, and that's all that's necessary.

Now look at the last column on your Pack Strap. Write the three highest numbers—when you smoke the most. Your stress periods should now be quite clear. Spend some time assessing those causes of excess smoking and decide what you can do instead. Repatterning is in order. For ideas, turn to "Tools to Cope" in the back of the book.

This is your last week of smoking! You are far better prepared than you realize. I know you wish you had done everything much more faithfully, but you can do it heart and soul this week, and have great success. Here's how:

- Honor the Delay Times faithfully, but distract yourself so you don't suffer.
- Do the oral gratification routine faithfully after each food intake.
- Record all cigarettes on the Pack Strap BEFORE you light up.
- Get enough rest, exercise, and eat lightly and often.
- Read your Reasons regularly; recite your five best several times a day. Write them on cards to remind you. WANT to quit so much that it hurts!
- When stress occurs, do the Relaxation Ritual (See Chapter 7).
- REWARD YOURSELF frequently—in little ways.
- Avoid self-pity at all costs.
- Maintain a positive attitude. You can do it, and you will. Over one million smokers have quit with this method—and many of them were heavier smokers, or smoked longer than you. YOU CAN DO IT!

Here are your instructions for the week:

1. Smoke as many as you like, but change your brand to any with .3 or less nicotine. (Refer to FTC chart at the back of the book.) *Buy enough for the week.* This will result in about a 92% reduction of nicotine intake compared to your former intake. Your detoxification has been effected gradually as a result of the reduction in the number of cigarettes smoked, the lower nicotine brands, and a variety of other techniques, such as increased water, exercise, etc.

So don't fear climbing the walls when you cut off. You won't.

2. Prepare the new Pack Strap, #4, in the back of the book. This time you will simply mark the time you have a cigarette, and then the reason. A reason may be an emotion, such as "angry" or "worried," or it could be "tired" or "hungry." You'll soon see that you don't have very many reasons to smoke anymore, and the only reason you smoke most of them is because you're allowed to before your Cut-Off date. That's okay too. Don't hold back now, and don't

Cut-Off prematurely. You set your Cut-Off date. You must honor it. If you cut-off sooner, you might feel you're "owed" a couple, and it will nag at you. Go the full mile to get the most out of this.

3. **Delay smoking for one hour** before bed and after ALL food and drink, except water, milk, juice, raw fruit and vegetables or boullion. This is the last delay time you'll have. After next week, you won't smoke so you won't have to delay!

4. **Repattern!** Don't sit and suffer until your hour is up. Get up from the table and do your oral gratification routine, then move to another area of interest not associated with smoking. For instance:

Don't sit in your favorite easy chair where you used to read the newspaper, or watch TV, and smoke. Instead go outside for a walk, or do some gardening, or fix the car or the porch light. It's a good idea to do things with your hands. Or take a shower . . . be creative.

5. **Don't smoke before breakfast.**

6. **Don't smoke while riding in a car.** If you feel like having one, pull off the road, get out and smoke. A good trick is to clean and polish your car on the inside today (a reward?) so it smells clean and fresh. After you quit smoking you'll resent people smoking in your car. It makes it stink. To give your smoking friends the word, graciously, put some artificial flowers in the ash tray.

7. **Don't smoke while talking on the telephone.** This will cut down on your phone bills. If the phone rings, don't light up. Talk. Hang up. Then you can smoke. You'll be surprised at how anxious you are to cut the call short. If you are a phone operator, or you do the bulk of your business on the phone, adapt the requirement so you gain the benefit of the instruction.

8. **Don't smoke while** typing, cooking, sewing, ironing, or any situation peculiar to your own lifestyle. If you always smoke when doing something, do it without smoking. When you're finished, walk away and light up.

9. Continue to **keep your cigarettes in an unfamiliar place**.

10. **Search your house, office, clothes pockets and purses for cigarettes.** Clean out any except your current supply. Don't leave any around to tempt you. This is an act of commitment. Sort of an "ending" ritual. Have fun doing it.

11. This week, **collect your butts for the week.** Use only one ash tray, if possible, but don't wipe out the ash tray all week. Put all the butts into a clear glass jar with a tight-fitting lid. You can bring the jar to the office, or bring the butts home in a baggie. I know this is gross, but it's the only evidence you will have of the filth related to smoking.

At the end of the week, after you've collected all you can, put a couple of drops of water in the jar and shake it up a bit. If ever you get an urge to smoke, you can open the jar and smell it. Or just look at it. It will "satisfy" your need.

I remember the day I "invented" the Butt Jar. It was my last week of smoking. I was at my desk, using a huge ash tray. The reason I used a huge one was because I hated to empty out ashtrays because of the dirt and the gook on the bottom of the ashtray, and little ones needed emptying very often. I was very conscious that I was smoking what might be my last few days. (If I sound morbid, that's how I felt. I really was afraid that I'd quit, and afraid that I wouldn't!) I thought, "I might never have to empty out another ash tray. These may be the last butts I'll ever create. Will I remember the dirtiness, and the gook on the bottom of the ash tray?" So I decided to put them in a mayonnaise jar and save them, in case I ever forgot. Now the Butt Jar is a standard in the SmokEnder program and even the Cancer Society has "borrowed" the idea for their program. Do it. It's useful.

When you finally wipe out the ash tray, remember that there's more gook on your lungs than there is on that ash tray—but in a short time, your body will cleanse itself and your lungs will be almost like those of a non-smoker (unless you have emphysema or cancer, which are in most cases irreversible).

12. **Prepare to save your smoking money.** Find a big glass jar with a screw top lid. Punch a slot in the lid so you can drop coins and bills into the jar. After you stop smoking, you will have a daily savings ritual. You'll find out about that next week.

Be ready to outsmart the habit this week. There is within you the same ambiguity that I felt. Your habit will try to survive by trying to get you to soften up on the delay times, or not recording each cigarette, or any of the other instructions. Be firm. Be confident that you want to be in control of your life—and not have cigarettes control you any more. Think about the importance of living a full and rich life right now. It's not a matter of dying a few years sooner. It's the quality of your life NOW. When you smoke, the quality is poorer.

Don't give in to the habit. You deserve to be free of it. You smoked long enough and paid dearly. You're worth the effort.

You're becoming eager and less afraid. In fact, you are probably anxious to be done with it. Your mind is responding to hope and increased self-worth.

You're working hard and doing a great job. Keep it up. I wish you the pleasure of NOT-SMOKING. You can do it.

Frequently during each day, and as you're falling asleep, recite your pledge:

I WILL STOP SMOKING
I WILL LOOK BETTER
I WILL FEEL BETTER
I WILL BE FREE!

WEEK FIVE

Tomorrow has the potential for being one of the most exciting days of your life.

You have prepared yourself in countless ways. You have essentially disconnected the circuitry that kept you a slave to cigarettes. From tomorrow on, you will be creating a new life-style for yourself. A much more satisfying, healthy and happy one, because you will be free of guilt (you aren't self-destructing anymore). And your body will become the efficient, vital organism it was meant to be before you started drugging it.

Review Pack Strap #4. Write the total in your notebook with the totals from previous weeks. No doubt the number of cigarettes is considerably lower than when you started this program. And the reasons for smoking are relatively meaningless. "Because I could" is probably the most stated reason.

It doesn't matter if you're still smoking a lot of cigarettes. The disconnecting has been going on in many other ways. Assuming you put a lot into this, you will get a lot out of it. *The single most important item is your desire to quit.* If you have built up your motivation so that you WANT TO QUIT more than anything else, you will quit successfully.

A few check points: be sure your main reasons are not to please someone else. For instance, if your main reason is to set a good example for your son, and then your son starts smoking pot or disappoints you in some way, your reason to stay off cigarettes will vanish in a stroke of SPITE. You'll say, "Look what I did for you, and you did this thing which hurts me!" So you start to smoke again. Two losers!

Also, be sure your main reason is not finite. For instance, "So I can have my physical next month and tell the doctor I don't smoke anymore." What happens the day after your check-up? Can you start to smoke then? Sure it feels great to say, "Doc, I quit smoking!" But that should not be a main reason.

Also, don't set yourself up to start again by saying, "I MUST quit because I have an ulcer (or some other health problem)." First of all, if you think you MUST quit, instead of feeling you WANT to quit, you'll resent the whole thing. You won't have the same quality of success. Find reasons that make quitting attractive to you. Also, if you MUST quit because of an ulcer, will you start smoking again when the ulcer is cured?

I have read thousands of follow-up questionnaires and letters from SmokEnder graduates and can spot candidates for relapse just by the quality and number of reasons they have. If they have only one or two, and those are MUST reasons, I fear for the longevity of their success in quitting. So work on your Reasons. Reread Chapter 12. Find reasons that really touch your heart and soul and make you WANT to quit.

Be sure you have enough cigarettes to smoke as many as you like—without running out of them before you're ready to quit.

When you run out of cigarettes tonight, or when you're ready for bed, whichever comes first, smoke your last cigarette.

Don't make a tragic farewell ceremony. You're getting rid of a big heavy monkey that has been on your back for a long time. You're trading it for freedom. It's a good deal.

And it's not negotiable.

When you take your last puff, drop it in the toilet or stub it out in your dirty ashtray—with finality. If you have any leftover cigarettes, drop them in the toilet or break them up and put them in the Butt Jar.

Here are your instructions for the week:

1. **Keep a Journal.** A written record of your days as a non-smoker. Each day in your notebook, write your feelings, successes, difficulties, accomplishments, whatever, so you can maintain control of your recovery. In this way, you can reread your journal and see how far you've come; what obstacles you licked; what successes have made you proud. The mind has a funny way of forgetting the pain and difficulty one endures.

Keeping a log of your journey becomes a vital reinforcement tool later on.

Start your log tonight. It might look something like this:

Today's date . . .

Tomorrow will be different. I won't be smoking. I can't believe it will happen, yet I somehow expect it will work. Wish I had done everything to the letter of the law, but I'm sure nobody could do everything exactly right, so I guess I'll be all right.

I smoked until two A.M. I thought I'd keep on smoking until I ran out of cigarettes, but it didn't seem too important, so I had my last one, threw it in the toilet, heaved a sigh of relief, which surprised me, and I'm off to bed.

Day One

Woke up this morning knowing something special was in the air. Then I remembered: I don't smoke anymore! I felt strangely elated. But apprehensive.

Got up, showered and dressed. No urges, but then I had done this many times before without a cigarette.

Had a good breakfast to keep my energy up all morning.

10 A.M. No urges yet. It feels unreal. I'm so conscious of everything happening around me. This must be that "heightened awareness" they talk about. I like it.

11:15 Ah-ha! I had a quick little desire for a cigarette when Jim came by with his coffee, but I realized it was both a conditional response and a bit of mid-morning "slump," so I took a little juice and a nice, deep breath. It passed. It was proud. It was so easy too.

3 P.M. This day is going a lot easier than I thought it would. I'm aware that I'm not smoking, but I don't want a cigarette. It's almost a detached feeling. I feel like I'm watching me. I'm not climbing the walls. I'm very comfortable but I'm afraid an urge will come that will be too hard to handle. . . .

10:30 P.M. This has been a remarkable day. I don't think I'll ever forget it. I feel so happy. And so "light" somehow. I feel very much in control of myself, yet I'm not really working at it. I had one or two small urges for a cigarette today, but the thought came and went before I could do anything about it. I wonder how it will go tomorrow . . .

P.S.: Nobody noticed that I wasn't smoking! And I thought everybody who has been nagging me to quit would be complimenting me, but they didn't notice!

This is an excerpt from a journal. It goes on in much the same manner for about four weeks. What is significant is that after the first few days, the new ex-smoker stabilizes and thinks he has it made. At that very time, he is hit with a desire for a cigarette that makes him rush to his notebook to find a distracting Reward. It happened again about three weeks after Cut-Off. But he didn't succumb. He liked being free and worked past it, using the techniques he learned in the program.

That's the critical time for you: about three days and three weeks after you quit. I suspect it happens because you take it for granted and your resolve softens, or you get cocky. Be on guard each day, and be grateful to be free at least.

Don't let it get away. Each night say to yourself, "It was a good day. I didn't smoke!"

3. To reinforce your new habit of not smoking, **begin a page in your notebook headed "Plusses."** Each day you'll notice nice things happening to you as a result of quitting. Write them down. Some are physical, some social, some emotional. For instance, you might discover that you don't have to clear your throat anymore; or you ask for non-smoking seats in the restaurant or airplane; you notice your eyes look clearer, less bloodshot; you run up the stairs without puffing. Write it down. You might discover that, because you've gained a great deal of self-confidence as a result of quitting smoking, you are more assertive in business or personal matters. So many good things happen when you quit smoking. The "Plusses" list is a very important self-reinforcing tool. Make it happen.

4. **Anticipate malice from your smoking friends and relatives.** Some may try to coax you to start smoking again. They won't believe you aren't suffering. Some may blow smoke in your face. Perhaps they're jealous that you could quit and they're still smoking, believing they can't quit. Or maybe they're afraid they'll be the last one in the board room or bridge club who smokes. They want you back in the fold!

5. **Paste little "cue cards" on your mirror** telling yourself how wonderful you are. "You're great. You don't smoke anymore!" Things like that. Celebrate your success. As you may discover, those people who seemed to be most concerned

about your smoking may not realize that you've quit. Don't count on them for reinforcement. They might even say, "Well, it's about time!" So build your own self-reinforcement.

6. Take the jar you prepared for your saving ritual and put it on top of your dresser next to your Butt Jar. **Each night drop in the amount of money you would have spent on cigarettes.** At this writing, cigarettes are between $2.00 and $2.50 a pack. So, if you smoked two packs a day, drop between $4.00 and $5.00 into the jar. Do this religiously. It's tangible evidence of your quitting smoking, *and* it builds up a nice sum for a big reward. Refer to the Cost of Smoking chart at the back of the book for the amount you'll save in a year. Put it in the bank each week or on the first of each month, and let it earn interest. It will really mount up. Plan that great vacation trip for a year from now. You can afford it. You've earned it!

If you're thinking you can't afford to save the money you're no longer spending on tobacco, let me tell you that if you continued to smoke, you would *find* the money somehow. That's the unfortunate truth about addiction.

To see what you have gained as a result of quitting, turn to the back of the book for sample charts showing how your smoking money compounds, over time at various interest rates. It's shocking!

7. Read your notebook from cover to cover tonight and refer to it during the weeks to come. Remember to continue doing those things which will aid you in maintaining success as a non-smoker. I know you're apprehensive about tomorrow morning. That's natural. But if you've done most of the activities required, and have an intense desire to be free, tomorrow has the potential for being one of the most exciting, awesome, joyous, surreal days of your life. Don't let fear hold you back—you're remarkably well-trained and ready to begin a new life—free of tobacco. Go for it!

Now change your recitation to present tense, and repeat it frequently:

> I DON'T SMOKE ANYMORE!
> I LOOK BETTER!
> I FEEL BETTER!
> I AM HAPPY!

15

What Happens After You Quit, and How to Stay Free Forever

CONGRATULATIONS! You have done something many millions of people wish they could do. You worked hard. You engaged your mind and body in the project, and you have achieved the result equal to your effort. You deserve to feel proud of yourself.

The next phase is the stabilizing phase. Your mind and body will be re-adjusting to your new non-smoking lifestyle. Don't feel you have it made. There are still many "disconnects" that must be made before you can consider yourself a non-smoker. At this stage, you are still an ex-smoker. Your old habit will try to outsmart you. You must constantly reinforce your desire to be free.

I hope your first weeks without cigarettes were a real high. I felt almost euphoric for a long time. The feeling of freedom, and the absence of a drug that slows you down combine to give many people a wonderful sense of elation. About 80% of all SmokEnder graduates report this "high."

Or you may not be feeling dramatically different—yet. For some people, it takes a little longer before the relief and freedom become real.

In either case, don't allow your freedom to disappear in one urge and one cigarette. I assure you, one cigarette leads to a pack, which leads to a carton. No matter who you are or how successful you've been.

HERE'S WHAT TO DO IN A PINCH: (Dog-ear this page so you can refer to it quickly.)

If you have an urge to smoke, first take one or two very deep breaths. (You used to take a deep drag when you smoked, so deep breathing is very satisfying now.)

Then, immediately say to yourself, "I don't smoke anymore. I don't want a cigarette, so what do I *really* want?" We call that "Decoding your Craving."

Then quickly do whatever it is that your mind or body is asking. We call that "distracting yourself." Refer to "Tools to Cope" in the back of the book.

• If you're hungry, eat.

• If your mouth is craving attention, brush and rinse or use a breath spray, or chew on a clove or ginger root.

• If you're tired, take a nap.

• If your energy is low, take some fructose or a small glass of orange or grapefruit juice, or hot bouillon.

• If you're angry, worried or disappointed, write in your journal or do something physical to let off steam.

• If you're bored, get up off your duff and make a reward happen for you and someone who needs some caring support.

• If you're feeling sorry for yourself, laugh at yourself and refer to your Rewards list for a quickie.

• If you're restless, change your locale and circumstances.

• If it's a "hidden trigger," recognize it as such, and put space between the condition and your former response. Be a good detective and identify hidden triggers BEFORE they occur so you're well prepared. (Hidden triggers are situations in which you smoked under circumstances that happened only occasionally, such as a funeral, hospital visit, coming back to your beach blanket after a swim, an accident, argument, annual visit to or from a cranky relative, etc.)

To protect yourself, refer to "Projecting Hidden Triggers" in back of book.

• If you're under great pressure, tense, or stressed, quickly do the Relaxation Ritual—or at least take a good deep breath until you can relax. Take a soothing warm bath. Refresh yourself: wash your face, comb your hair, and drink a nice cold glass of water.

• If you're having a physical discomfort—a "Symptom of Recovery"—refer to the chart at the back of the book for recommendations.

• If the urge becomes a craving, recite your five best reasons for wanting to be a non-smoker; open the Butt Jar and take a whiff.

• If you have a buddy, call him or her. Even if they aren't in, the act of calling is often distraction enough, because . . .

EVEN IF YOU DO NOTHING ABOUT THE URGE, IT WILL PASS IN A FEW SECONDS. DISTRACTING JUST PUTS YOU IN CONTROL.

After you have quit smoking for a week or two, it is helpful to tell a few of your closest friends and relatives and enlist their support. Say something like this: "For the past several weeks I've put myself through a rigorous program to break my smoking habit. I'm pleased to say I haven't smoked in X weeks, and I'm determined to stay off. However, the smoking habit is very tenacious, and it will be some time before I can feel safe from relapse. You can help me in several ways. If I succumb to any one of a hundred lures to have a cigarette, and ask you for one, saying 'One won't hurt,' or 'I can handle it,' don't give it to me. Tell me to go over my reasons for wanting to quit, or my plusses. Or remind me how you care for me and don't want me to get sick or depart prematurely. Then help distract me by suggesting we change what we're doing, where we are. . . ."

If the urge strikes, call one of those people with whom you shared your feelings, and tell them you need their support.

• Until you're stabilized in your new habit of not-smoking, put another sign on your mirror and on your desk that says, "One will hurt." If your resolve begins to falter and you consider taking a cigarette, declare to yourself: *"It's not negotiable. I have no options. I've quit."*

• To increase your motivation to stay quit, you must constantly reinforce yourself for the first few months. Therefore, as you discover new reasons why you're glad you quit, write those reasons in your workbook and on little cards—one per card—and put them in highly visible places: on the mirror in your bathroom, on the windshield of your car, on your desk, and so on. Be on the constant lookout for added reasons why you enjoy not-smoking.

There are many subtle reasons which will emerge over a long period of time if you keep alert for them. For instance, many months after I quit smoking, I realized my eyelids didn't burn when I awoke in the morning. It used to be so difficult to open my eyes—my eyelids felt like sandpaper. When I quit smoking, the scratchiness disappeared. Coincidence? No. Apparently the smoke had caused a chronic subclinical irritation.

Another discovery after I quit smoking: for years when our children were young I'd sing to them and accompany myself on the guitar. When our oldest child, Joan, became big enough to manage a guitar, we sang and played together frequently. Even as a small child she had a good ear and a lovely voice. It was a pleasure we all enjoyed. But our little concerts became shorter and shorter because my throat began to pain me after a short round of singing. I suppose deep down I suspected a relationship between the pain and my smoking, but I didn't mention it. How could I indict my beloved buddy? By that time, my family had begun their campaign to get me to quit smoking. So I made excuses, and Joan sang without me. After a few years I stopped singing altogether. Joan went on to become the family songmistress; but we had all loved to sing when we were together, and I regretted no longer being able to take part. It was a pleasure denied. Looking back, I think it was probably my first truly personal reason for wanting to quit smoking. The discovery, years later, that I could sing without discomfort—and, as a bonus, that my voice became clearer and not so deep—was a strongly reinforcing surprise reason.

One woman wrote to tell me she was glad she quit smoking because people don't call her "sir" on the phone anymore.

Don't take your freedom for granted. Reinforce yourself at every opportunity. Search for reasons why you're glad you don't smoke anymore.

See Chapter 16, "Why You're Glad You Quit Smoking." It will help you add some profound, amusing, and clearly important reasons.

• Now create a clean, fresh, non-smoking environment around yourself. Surround yourself with non-smokers. Now that smoking is banned in most indoor workplaces—or soon will be (it is expected that OSHA will ban smoking in ALL workplaces in the U.S.) it will be easier to stay "clean" because cigarettes and smokers won't be in evidence. Won't it be nice not to have to go outside in the cold to get a fix anymore? Rejoice!

• Another trap for many ex-smokers is self-pity. If you should happen to feel sorry for yourself for any reason— don't reach for a cigarette. Laugh at yourself for being childish, and say to yourself, "*Smoking won't make anything better*. What is it I really want?"

• After you quit, don't abuse your friends with your self-righteousness or hassle them about their smoking. Rather, tell them how well you feel now that you don't smoke anymore. It's very reinforcing to tell others how much energy and vitality you now feel. For instance, it's more helpful to yourself and your smoking friend to say, "Since I quit smoking I can jog a couple of miles" or "play two more sets of tennis before wearing down" or "run up the stairs without becoming winded." Your friends will applaud you instead of avoiding you. And you might save a life, because your friend might take interest in quitting because you made it seem so desirable and pleasurable.

And you can reinforce yourself by creating a local non-smoking epidemic among your friends, business associates, colleagues, relatives. Your example will certainly infect others. People will say, "If you could quit smoking, I can." Encourage people to quit for the *pleasure* of not-smoking. It's a strange new concept. And it's real.

Now that you did it, you can help others with this book. Begin a group in your home, office or club—or help someone one-on-one. Inquire about the "Facilitator's Guide," which spells out the procedure clearly.

• Finally, each month, on your anniversary of quitting, plan a really fine celebration. Take yourself out to dinner, to the theater or to a sporting event—or buy yourself something special on that date with the money you saved. (See Cost of Smoking chart.) It will become as important and remembered as your birthday—and in fact, it might well be. For many of us, it is the day we really began to live as free people.

As you move about in the world as a non-smoker, you will encounter traps and hazards that could give you an excuse to resume smoking. If you know where they lie, you can circumvent them.

Here are the danger signs to watch for. Study this list. Read it frequently, until you know it by heart:

"SANDTRAPS"
(OR HOW TO AVOID THE MOST FREQUENT CAUSES OF RECIDIVISM)

1. COMPLACENCY
One quickly forgets the discomforts of smoking . . . the difficulty of quitting. The mind has a convenient memory and remembers only the good.

A smoker may con himself into believing that he's "got it made." Once past the direct activity of quitting, it's easy to say "one won't hurt" and then, according to reports, somehow, over the weeks, "one" has become "one pack a day!" *One chink in the wall of your resolve begins erosion of the wall.* A study several years ago by Dr. Donald T. Fredrickson, then of the N.Y. City Board of Health, revealed that 15 out of 25 recidivists resumed smoking because of complacency.

Don't ever take for granted your hard-earned freedom!

2. ALCOHOL (AND/OR "GRASS")
A manifestation of complacency, nothing softens the resolve like alcohol. The danger is not the cocktail party as a

trigger situation but that *marginal excess which strips you of control* and allows rationalizations to swarm. The "high" when one is apt to say, "What the hell . . . I won't worry about it tonight." Avoid heavy drinking (and pot parties) until you have stabilized your attitude and begun to enjoy not smoking.

3. WEIGHT

Those people who view quitting smoking as a form of self-denial and reach for food as a substitute, are creating an excuse to start again. An increase in weight is viewed by the mature person as another challenge or project which will be managed at the right time. *Weight*, in itself, *does not create cravings for a cigarette.* All too often we hear that people who resume smoking because they gained weight find themselves *saddled with the double problem of being overweight smokers.*

4. PHYSIOLOGICAL PROBLEMS

Individuals who have become impatient with a sometimes *lingering Symptom of Recovery*—such as muddle-headedness, drowsiness, constipation—forget that they are temporary and *transient*. Consider how long and much one smoked—everything cannot disappear overnight. BE PATIENT. *The body will restore itself. Keep perspective. Is the danger and misery of the smoking habit a fair trade-off for one annoying Symptom of Recovery?*

5. PERSONAL PROBLEMS

We will always be distressed with personal problems. Life is like that. *To smoke in the face of a personal problem is counterproductive.* THERE ARE NO REASONS FOR SMOKING . . . ONLY EXCUSES. Remember, SMOKING NEVER MADE ANYTHING BETTER.

6. "MY MATE/BUDDY/LOVER/WHOEVER STARTED"

A person with whom you share your life has started smoking. "It's not fair," or "Cigarettes are always around now," etc. Would you use that person's toothbrush? Then don't smoke that person's cigarettes—they're not yours. We are all free to make our own choices. You have chosen not to smoke. It's your choice to be free.

7. REATTRACTED AND/OR TASTE

"Smoking never lost its charm" is what this type tells us. Do you recognize any *self-deception* in that one? Or, "I just wanted to see how it tasted," or, "I missed the taste." Too bad! We agreed cigarettes taste lousy.

8. BOREDOM

Evidence of boredom being a key factor in smoking was shown in the old cigarette commercials, "Me and my Winston" or "This is the L&M Moment." For many people (not just widows or elderly people who are alone) *loneliness and boredom* are the core of their universe. A cigarette becomes their only friend and the *only sparkle of life and excitement that they seem to be able to generate for themselves*. The tragedy is that in this busy world, which *needs* human contribution, only the bedridden might be forgiven for being bored. So . . . set new goals and make the most of yourself—not the least. Improve yourself with new skills and knowledge. Make yourself important to other people. Become involved.

9. SPITE

When pressures pile up . . . the world seems against you, the boss is impossible, the spouse or kids for whom you quit give you a hard time, a natural reaction is: "I'll show him (her/them) . . . I'll have a cigarette. Look at the sacrifice I made in quitting and this is the thanks I get . . . I'll smoke one just for spite!" TO SPITE WHO? Case histories show this *spirals down* to a big case of "poor me" and results in *self-pity cycle*. This is one of the prime reasons for insisting you have a sincere *personal* desire to quit—not for your family or someone else.

10. IGNORANCE IN SWITCHING

Smokers like to persuade themselves that there are "safe" cigarettes . . . "less hazardous" pipes or cigars. SmokEnders graduates know that this is simply *not true*. Dr. Alton Ochsner, when asked about the safety of other forms of smoking, replied: "It remains with the smoker to choose the site of his cancer"; that is, ANY CIGARETTE OR TOBACCO PRODUCT IS SAFE UNTIL YOU PUT IT IN YOUR MOUTH!

11. COMPLETION OF THE PLEASURABLE CYCLE

Here is a specific application of complacency at work under totally *non-threatening,* comfortable circumstances.

When one has finished a particularly good and pleasant meal; when one has enjoyed an afternoon or evening of pleasant activity; when one is surrounded by good friends (who may or may not be smoking), etc., one has a sudden feeling of wanting to do that ''one more thing'' to make the whole situation perfect—*the Completion of the Pleasurable Cycle.*

It isn't the automobile accident or the argument with the boss or teenage son or the sudden, acute business problem that is the culprit—but, rather, a comfortable, pleasant occasion during which one feels no real concern.

The most important thing to remember is that pleasurable events cannot be enhanced by smoking—rather they will be marred by the guilt and anger you'll feel for lighting up.

12. THE LACK OF SELF-WORTH

For the one who has developed self-confidence and a strong sense of self-worth as a result of quitting smoking, the chances of *starting again are very slim.* He gets to know himself finally as an adult, accepts his limitations and strengths, feels comfortable with himself, and doesn't need to make excuses for his actions any longer. He has achieved *something of value . . .* has earned his *own respect!* This is *maturity,* which is based on self-respect. To such a person, the thought of taking a cigarette *represents the loss of personal dignity and freedom.* Viktor E. Frankl, writing of his concentration camp experience, wrote in his book, *Man's Search For Meaning*:

> Everything can be taken away from a man but one thing:
> The last of the Human Freedoms—to choose one's attitude in
> any given set of circumstances—to choose one's own way!

CHOOSE TO ENJOY NOT SMOKING!

Each of the above listed causes of recidivism is a possible chink in the crack of your armor. Any one, if it finds a tiny crack, will break through and cause your new freedom some real problems.

When your reason(s) to be free of the habit are strong—your MOTIVATION is your armor. NOTHING can penetrate it—no seductive memory of your lost "love" . . . no stressful situation . . . no complacency . . . NOTHING!

When the benefits and pleasure of not-smoking exceed any benefit or pleasure you thought smoking gave you, you will be truly free. That's why those of us who are happily liberated are confident we'd never want to smoke again. We'd feel like we were losing something of great value. It's such a pleasure not to smoke.

So—the secret of success is building onto your Reasons for being glad you don't smoke anymore—strengthening your MOTIVATION—every day at every opportunity. Then nothing can ever make you take that first cigarette.

16

Why You're Glad You Quit Smoking

Now I can talk to you as a "member of the club." The ex-smoker's club. It's a wonderful club. Membership brings you additional free benefits: More money for you—instead of for the tobacco club; the ability to see clearly—the propaganda put out by the tobacco industry; the freedom from worry and guilt that you're hurting yourself and others; the absence of excuses for your inability to control your own life; and a good feeling about yourself.

During the twenty-two years I was desperately trying to quit smoking, I was assaulted with health facts: horrific details about the terrible things that would happen to me if I continued to smoke. That was called "scare tactics." The reasoning was that if I knew how bad smoking was—and the consequences—I would surely quit.

Alas, it worked in reverse. The worse the news, the more I smoked. Obviously, it didn't work for me. And it doesn't seem to work for the majority of smokers. After all, is there a smoker over sixteen who doesn't know the hazards of smoking and the gruesome potential for misery and premature death? And yet, knowing the worst, most continue to smoke . . .

As for me, I didn't want to hear or know anything about smoking—while I smoked. I didn't want to hear any health facts or anything negative about smoking. I was a very defensive smoker. I even defended the tobacco industry when I was pressed! They were my "suppliers"—and so my benefactors.

So I skirted the "fear tactics" when I worked out a method for me to quit. I knew scare tactics were counterproductive. It was like beating a dead horse. Instead, I focused on the positive aspects of quitting. As you read in the book, I built in frequent rewards, satisfactions, indulgences. I focused on "What's in it for me." I looked forward to the joy of having that monkey off my back. I set freedom and self-mastery as my goal, instead of self-preservation.

It was not until after I quit that I began to see the peril of smoking with new eyes. Health information now became hugely reinforcing. I was relieved to know that I had moved to the safer side of my behavior—and that I would be able to put the worry and guilt behind me.

And now it's different for you too. Now that you quit, you can look at the whole subject of smoking with new eyes. It will become fascinating, as you move away from your addiction.

Now I bring you the facts as a form of reinforcement. While reading what follows, consciously allow your mind to recite an "affirmation" to acknowledge your freedom. Something like, "Thank the powers that be/God/the Universe (or whatever you thank) I don't smoke anymore and that I don't have to carry the burden and worry that smoking causes. I'm glad I'm FREE!"

Here, then, are some oddments and facts for starters. Items that will make you glad you quit when you did:

• Smokers are not only more prone to duodenal ulcers, but smoking leads to slower healing rates and greater recurrence. Happily, now that you've stopped smoking, the chances of ulcer are dramatically reduced.

• Now that you quit you're saving approximately one tree every two weeks. That's what it takes, per smoker, to cure the tobacco. (Curing tobacco is one of the greatest single demands for wood.)

• To pay for smoking-related illnesses, each non-smoking, working-age adult in the United States pays in excess of $100 a year extra in taxes and health insurance premiums. By quitting, you have lowered that cost.[1]

• Cigarettes cause about 65,000 fires a year in the United States, resulting in $300 million in property damage, 2,300 deaths and 5,000 injuries. Smoking-related fires kill more people than any other kind of fire.[2]

• Annually, smoking irritants contribute to the 1.8 million reported cases of sinusitis, which develop about 75% more often in smokers. When you quit smoking, the sinusitis symptoms usually disappear.[3]

• Lung cancer is the principal cause of cancer deaths for both sexes, and smoking accounts for approximately 87% of lung cancer deaths. Many of the remaining 13% of lung cancers are now thought to be caused by secondhand/passive smoking.[4]

• If you're French you won't be contributing to the three tons of butts collected as garbage every day in the Paris Metro.[5]

• And if you're an American, you won't be adding to the beach litter: 1,700,000 cigarette butts collected after a holiday weekend on a public beach on Long Island, New York— the biggest load of *ALL* litter! If placed end to end they would reach 27 miles. UGH.

• Cigar or pipe use increases the risk for cancers of the lung, mouth, throat, larynx and esophagus.[6]

• In 1985, an estimated 390,000 people died from smoking-related diseases. By 1988, it increased to 434,000. A calculation was made to determine the number of potential life-years lost by smokers who died from smoking-related diseases before age sixty-five—an astonishing 1,198,887 years! During 1990, the number of smoking-related deaths increased to 418,690—approximately 20% of ALL deaths. That's almost 1,200 smokers a day.

• The following smoking-attributable deaths for 1990:

- Sudden Infant Death Syndrome, believed to be related to secondhand smoke: 470
- Burn deaths caused by smoking: 1,362.
- Urinary cancers (bladder, kidney, other urinary): 7,200
- Pancreatic cancer attributable to smoking: 6,114
- Respiratory diseases, including emphysema: 84,475
- Pediatric diseases (other than Sudden Infant Death): 1,241
- Cardiovascular diseases: 179,820
- Cancers, all: 145,631[7]

• Since 1950, 2,494,000 people died of lung cancer. It is estimated that 87% of lung cancer deaths were caused by smoking; therefore, 2,169,780 people: mothers and fathers, sisters and brothers, aunts and uncles, sons and daughters—real people—suffered and died unnecessarily. Prematurely. Now that you have quit, your body has begun to restore itself, so that over time your risk diminishes almost to that of a non-smoker.

• Out of $87 billion spent by Medicare on in-patient hospital care this year, at least $20 billion is due to substance abuse: 80% due to smoking, 3% to drug abuse, and 17% to alcohol abuse, according to Joseph A. Califano, Jr., head of Columbia University's Center on Addiction and Substance Abuse. "Substance abuse will cost Medicare $1 trillion for hospital care over the next twenty years—and smoking will be responsible for most of it."[8]

• R.J. Reynolds, Jr., son of the founder of the tobacco company that bears his name, died at age fifty-eight from emphysema. His son, R.J. Reynolds III, half brother of Patrick, died at age sixty in 1994, of emphysema and congestive heart failure after a lifetime of cigarette smoking. Patrick Reynolds, grandson of RJR, Jr., and half brother of RJR III, is an anti-smoking campaigner and founder of Citizens for a Smoke-free America.[9]

• You won't be as likely to have an automobile accident now that you quit. Studies show that many accidents are due to drivers who were groping for their dropped, lit cigarette. Has it ever happened to you? It did to me. The cigarette would stick on my lips as I removed it after a puff—and flip away.

• Cataracts: As a smoker, your chances of getting cataracts were 50% to 60% greater than non-smokers. BUT, now that you have quit, the risk is greatly reduced.[10]

• Because you quit, you'll be less likely to land in the hospital: One-third of all hospital beds are devoted to tobacco-caused disease.[11] The annual medical tab for smokers is $50 billion. Half the money is spent on hospitalization alone.

• Because you quit, if you ever need orthopedic surgery, your bones will heal more quickly and you'll have less complications than if you continued to smoke.[12]

• If you're a woman, you have reduced your risk of cervical cancer and several complications of pregnancy, including bleeding during pregnancy, premature rupture of membranes, preterm delivery, placenta previa, abruptio placenta and low birth weight, because you quit smoking. If you're pregnant and stop smoking during the first trimester, the risk is reversed.[13]

• Cigarette companies spent $5,232,917,000 (billion) in 1992 for advertising and promotion. That comes to something like $6,000 AN HOUR!

• "Smoking has become associated with lower educational attainment and lower social status," says Dr. Jonathan Fielding, professor of Public Health, UCLA, and former Commissioner of Health.

• The Environmental Protection Agency classified secondhand smoke as a Group A carcinogen. Secondhand smoke kills 53,000 Americans every year. Not only are you saving your own life by quitting—you may be saving the lives of those around you.

• The tobacco industry is a $40 billion-plus-a-year business. Subtract the amount you smoked per year—plus the amount that over 30 million smokers who have quit or died in the last twenty years or so. It adds up. That's why they seek to entice new smokers—even children—to fill the gap of those smokers who quit or died. They spent $5,231,917 in 1992 to replace lost smokers.

They need someone to smoke an average of 10,128 cigarettes a year—that's about 500 packs. And at a soon to be average four dollars per pack, that's $2,000 a year per new customer. (The basis of these facts: In 1992, Americans smoked 506,400,000,000 (That's BILLION) cigarettes, or 2,675 cigarettes for each man and woman over eighteen in the U.S. But since there are only fifty million smokers left, each must smoke 10,128 cigarettes a year.)

• Now that you don't smoke anymore, you may not have to worry about being refused a job if you live in New Jersey. Legislators have been attempting to pass a law allowing employers to refuse to employ smokers. The pro-smoking tobacco lobby says people have a right to smoke—but, as Regina Carlson, New Jersey director of GASP (Group Against Smoking Pollution) says so cleverly, "Smoking is no more a civil right than being overweight."

I think it's less of a "right" than being overweight. Some people are born with a genetic disposition to carry more weight. A better comparison would be something of choice— perhaps, "Smoking is no more a right than choosing to wear blue clothes."

We chose to smoke (although we did not choose to get addicted). Rights are protected for those things we don't choose: like our sex, age, and color.

• As a non-smoker, you won't inhale and collect a half cup (or more) tar. "Tar" includes hydrogen *cyanide* and nitrogen dioxide and more than 600 chemical additives!

• The tobacco industry is accused of lying to the public. They knew nicotine was addictive in the fifties but hid the research.[14]

• Studies now show that smoking does not enhance creativity or complex calculations. The brain needs oxygen to function efficiently; instead, smoke from the cigarette converts pure oxygen into carbon monoxide, so it loses the ability to function at peak performance. More carbon monoxide is inhaled by smoking a pack of cigarettes than by breathing carbon monoxide gas fumes from directly behind your car. The effect is not lethal because it isn't concentrated, due to the time span required to smoke a cigarette.

• Smoking doesn't improve judgment and performance, either. A study by George Spilich of Washington College, Chestertown, Maryland, demonstrated that while smokers and non-smokers performed almost the same on simple, monotonous tasks, in complex tasks, like driving, smokers did poorly. For instance, smokers were involved in almost three times as many rear-end collisions as non-smokers in the group. He determined that drivers driving, pilots piloting, and others performing complex and important tasks, will probably not perform optimally if they smoke while they work. (Author's note: They have difficulty with judgment and performance when they quit cold-turkey, too. I hope I don't get a pilot who is trying to quit.)

• Tobacco leaves are sticky—like petunia leaves. Everything that passes by adheres to them. Bugs, worms, pesticides, fallout from the sky, dust, mud splashes from the rain, whatever. The leaves are hung to dry and "cured." And then processed, ground up. Nicotine is extracted and replaced in quantities necessary for the brand—plus thousands of additives: chemicals, flavorings, etc., and finally packed into the little white cylinders for us to smoke.

Can you imagine what you're really smoking? It was the idea of inhaling dead bugs that got me.

The process of reconstituting the tobacco allows the tobacco manufacturer to use the cheap blend of scraps, stems, dust, etc., instead of the more costly tobacco—and still provide desirable levels of nicotine.[15]

Tobacco farmers are furious because there is less demand for their crops. What does that do to the tobacco industry's argument that tobacco regulation and restrictions will be hard on tobacco farmers? They obviously don't really care about the farmers.

• To the argument that smoking doesn't cause cancer: The incidence of lung cancer among women increased 400% since 1950, when women started smoking in great numbers. In 1986 it surpassed breast cancer as the leading cause of death among women. Cancer has a long, slow fuse. It takes about twenty to thirty years to show up. A graph of the number of women smoking at each decade, and the number of cases of lung cancer among women, would show a parallel increase—but about twenty years apart. So much for the argument about whether or not smoking causes cancer.

• Smoking kills over 400,000 Americans each year—more than alcohol, homicide, cocaine, crack, heroin, fires, automobile accidents and AIDS combined!

• Smoking is the greatest cause of death and disability in the United States. That places a huge burden on health care costs. One solution: To tax tobacco. Here's how the numbers work out: There are fifty million smokers in the U.S. × number of packs smoked/day × 1.5 = total packs smoked/day, or 75 million.

• If the new tax were only a dollar per pack, that's $75 million dollars a DAY for health care. Over $27 BILLION per year. Not only does it raise money for health care—it reduces the cost of health care (because more people quit smoking for COST than almost anything else). Yes, there will be a proportionate reduction in the tax collected—but the net result is positive for non-smoking citizens. Many countries are taking the lead in this proposal. Cigarettes in Canada cost six dollars as of this writing, and the number of smokers has dropped significantly.

Now for a big horse laugh.

The results of a study were announced quite seriously, although I think they must be kidding. The study found that smoking helps keep health care costs down—it saves taxpayers money because *smokers die early so they don't incur all the medical costs attributable to aging—largely supported by Medicare.*[16]

P.S.: Guess who funded the study? One of the large tobacco companies.

What strikes my funny bone is, first, they admit that smoking kills you, and second, it kills you when you're young. By their reasoning, we ought to give everyone assault weapons so more people could shoot each other. That, too, would cut health care costs, wouldn't it? What they don't mention is that smoking costs and costs and costs—UNTIL the person dies. Younger or older. Smokers don't just up and die one day. They linger. They need medical care, medications, hospital care, usually surgery, and other manner of treatment.

I hope they didn't pay too much for that study.

• Young growing tissues are much more susceptible to carcinogens than adult tissues are. Bringing up a child in a smoking household is tantamount to bringing him or her up in a house lined with asbestos and radon.[17]

• The good news: Kids aren't as gullible as they were. In 1976, almost 29% of high school seniors smoked every day. By 1990, that number dropped to around 16%. In fact, smoking is falling among adults, too. Smoking peaked at 42% in 1964, the year the Surgeon General first reported that smoking caused cancer. Now only 26% of adults (people over eighteen) smoke.[18]

• Smoking doesn't necessarily kill you quickly. It more often MAIMS the smoker. For instance, the heart of a smoker beats 10,000 more times a day than a non-smoker. No wonder there are so many heart conditions caused by smoking.

From *Kids Say Don't Smoke*:
If you're ever going to have a baby you won't have to worry as much about Sudden Infant Death Syndrome (SIDS) if you don't smoke. A Swedish study found that light smokers were twice as likely as non-smokers to lose their babies to SIDS. Heavy smokers (ten cigarettes or more a day) were three times as likely.

Author's note: Someone should study the relationship between SIDS and fathers who smoke.

Also, low birth weight has been conclusively linked to cigarette smoking during pregnancy.[19]

• In 1990, children under eighteen bought cigarettes from vending machines on the order of 450,000 times a day.[20]

What can you do to eliminate this source of purchase by youngsters? Until the federal government restricts use of vending machines, it's a local and state matter. Call your mayor and municipal officers. Express your desire to eliminate vending machines. Write to your state representatives and your federal congressperson and senators. It really matters. If you can motivate your child to write to these lawmakers, it will be impressive, and provide a good civics lesson and a positive imprint upon their minds.

• A prominent heart surgeon told Larry King, the radio and TV personality, that "if everyone stopped smoking today, more than one-third of all the hospitals in the country would close in the next five years!"

• PASSIVE SMOKING kills 50,000 Americans a year—as many as died in the entire Vietnam War. Two-thirds died of heart disease. So your smoking was killing your family and your co-workers. Good you stopped or you'd be a candidate for homicide.

• Something to make you angry: When a tobacco company executive was asked why he didn't smoke, he answered, "Are you kidding? We reserve that right for the young, the poor, the black and the stupid."[21]

• Although Europeans and Asians are joining the war on smoking, the tobacco industry is vigorously promoting smoking in developing countries—to ensure their profitability.[22] It is embarrassing to Americans to see that we're exporting disease and premature death.
In China, 70% of men smoke. American cigarette manufacturers market heavily in such countries to make up for ailing U.S. demand by seeking new markets overseas.[23]

• You can breathe a sigh of relief and stop worrying that you might set your house on fire with a forgotten lit cigarette—or because you fall asleep watching TV or reading with a cigarette in your hand. Over 1,500 people die each year from cigarette-caused fires—the leading cause of fire deaths in houses, apartments, hotels, motels and mobile homes.

• Now that you're on the "rational" side of smoking, and you want to take action and support those who are working hard to overtake the power of the cigarette industry, here are some good organizations. I suggest you write for information and join if you can:

Americans for Nonsmokers' Rights
2530 San Pablo Avenue
Berkeley, CA 94702
   A national advocacy group protecting non-smokers from involuntary smoking. Publishes "ANR Update." Contains great information and news on local, state and federal efforts.

ASH: Action on Smoking and Health
2013 H. St. NW
Washington, DC 20006
   The legal arm of the fight. John Banzhalf, a lawyer and professor of law at Georgetown University, is a pioneer in the anti-smoking campaign. He single handedly caused cigarette ads to be banned from TV, and other noteworthy successes.

STAT: Stop Teenage Addiction to Tobacco
121 Lyman St #210
Springfield, MA 01103
   Publishes *Tobacco and Youth Reporter*. A must if you have children.

DOC: Doctors Ought to Care
1423 Harper Street
Augusta, GA 30912
   The good guys—they put their money where their mouths are.

NOTES

1. K.E. Warner, University of Michigan School of Public Health.
2. Joan Beck, *Chicago Tribune*, April 23, 1994.
3. Dental Teamwork, 1989
4. Center for Disease Control, Report of the Surgeon General, 1989.
5. *Time* magazine, April 18, 1994.
6. Center for Disease Control, "Reducing the health consequences of smoking," Report of the Surgeon General, 1989
7. Center for Disease Control, "Table of relative risks," August 27, 1993.
8. *The New York Times*, May 18, 1994.

9. *Time* magazine, July 25, 1994.
10. *Time* magazine, September 7, 1992.
11. Andrew Tobias, *Time* magazine, October 12, 1992.
12. Academy of Orthopedic Surgery, based upon research done by Emery School of Medicine.
13. *Tobacco and the Clinician*, National Institute of Health, 1994
14. Knight Ridder, May 18, 1994.
15. *Tobacco Free Youth Reporter*, Summer 1994.
16. Monitor Radio, September 2, 1994.
17. Dr. William G. Cahan, Surgeon, Memorial Sloan-Kettering Cancer Center.
18. *Kids Say Don't Smoke*, Andrew Tobias, Workman Publishing.
19. Ibid.
20. Ibid.
21. David Goerlitz, former cigarette model, ibid.
22. *Time* magazine, November 23, 1992.
23. *Time* magazine, June 1, 1992.

A Final Note from Jackie

Congratulations to you for having come this far.

I know that most people who read this book will benefit. Some will stop smoking—happily and permanently; some will be motivated to begin the process in earnest; some, who quit earlier or who are on the patch or gum, will have gained understanding and comfort; while some will want more direct participation and supervision, as in the SmokEnders Seminar.

At this writing, public seminars are available only in several major cities in this country and abroad. In-house seminars are conducted on the premises of large companies and organizations, but are generally not open to the public. However, there is now a superb and complete audiocassette program that simulates the actual seminar environment. It can be used for one person—or, with extra workbooks, for a group.

In addition, if you feel you need a group, and would like to put one together using this book, write for information about the "Facilitator's Guide." It's an old axiom that you help yourself when you help others. It's also gratifying—if you help someone stop smoking, it's as if you saved a life.

Now that it's no longer necessary for me to manage SmokEnders, I have been working to create several other projects, once again dealing with my own frailties as well as the experience of working with thousands of smokers.

Over the years, people have urged me to "do what I did for smokers" for other problems. So I have been working on DietEnders (because I carried too much weight, but wanted to lose it healthily), FatiguEnders (because I endured Chronic Fatigue Syndrome for four years and conquered it!), CaffeinEnders (because I shook off a heavy-duty coffee and Diet Coke habit), and SpenderEnders (what can I say?).

I expect they will be available in book or pamphlet form soon. They're all based upon the same principles as SmokEnders: a positive unlearning, relearning, detox from an addictive substance or emotional stimulant; rewards, self-knowledge and maximum motivational development, etc.

In this book I've mentioned several products I find valuable to help people stop smoking, such as Meal-In-A-Bag®, fructose tablets, and EnergyTabs. I'm attempting to find product people who can meet my standards of quality and make those products available.

☐ If you'd like further information about SmokEnders—for yourself or your company, or the audiocassette program, call:

> SmokEnders International 1-800-828-4357

☐ If you want information about the vitamin product I recommend, ALL-1, call:

> 1-800-235-5727, ext. 95

☐ If you'd like to be informed when other products, programs and my motivational and reinforcement tapes will be available, send me a note:

> Jacquelyn Rogers
> Box 550
> Easton, PA 18044-0550

Now I'd like to ask a favor: I would love to hear from you. Let me know how you did—what worked especially well, what didn't or what could. There's a questionnaire at the end of the book for your convenience. Although I can't respond to *all* my mail, please know that I am most grateful for your effort. Your input helps us help others more effectively.

To thank you, here's a toast:

• Here's to a world in which ashtrays are used to hold flower pots but never again for ashes . . .

• Here's to the day when our children are empowered to choose good health instead of being seduced and manipulated to become addicted to tobacco (and other things) . . .

• Here's to the day when legislators never again need to

feel pressured by tobacco interests—*because there is simply no market for tobacco* . . .

• Here's to the day when health care costs go DOWN because there are one-third less hospital beds and medical care required than when people smoked . . .

• And to the day when good people don't suffer and die, needlessly, painfully, prematurely, from tobacco . . .

• Here's to this great planet, which will have a cleaner and healthier environment without smoke and butts from billions of cigarettes a day . . .

• And, finally, here's to you—for working to free yourself from a wretched old buddy that was trying to kill you and was costing you a fortune.

By quitting, you are helping to make it all happen.

Now I want to talk to you about my personal challenge: Since 1969, when I was liberated from my seemingly hopeless enslavement to cigarettes, I vowed to do my best to create a non-smoking epidemic in this country. I knew it could be done, because I witnessed the disappearance of spittoons, which were everywhere when I was a child. Public opinion and an educated populace wiped them out. Now it's happening to smoking. And you are part of it. You have stopped paying dues in the tobacco "club"; you're on the "right" side of the tobacco issue.

While we smoke, and feel helpless in our addiction, we don't want to admit that the cigarette companies are selling sickness and death. We don't want to see it that way. In fact, we're defensive when people suggest we attack the tobacco industry.

I was defensive too, while I was helplessly entangled in the smoking web, but since I've been "liberated" I have seen the damage done by tobacco.

I've seen a young mother, in her forties, suddenly struck down with lung cancer. Killed, you could say. She had smoked for about twenty years—then, within six months of her diagnosis, she was gone. Her children, a little girl of ten and a sensitive son of thirteen, were heartbroken. I was angry. You see, her death was unnecessary. If she didn't smoke, she would not have died so young.

I've seen many men and women who look much older

than they are, because they're struggling to breathe. They paid their dues to the tobacco industry—for too many years. Emphysema is, in many ways, worse than cancer. It doesn't kill quickly. It just suffocates the victim—over long years, until their hearts give out.

I've seen the tragedy of a beloved husband cut down in his early fifties. He was my favorite brother-in-law, and good smoking buddy. He and my sister were lovebirds since they were in high school. Just when their three daughters were out on their own, and their lives could have become their own again, he suffered a massive heart attack. The first of three within a year and a half. His two and a half packs a day of Luckys got him. What was particularly rough was his inability to resist the craving for cigarettes. An added agony. He was damned if he smoked and damned if he didn't.

Sure, he cut down. He couldn't smoke around my sister, and since he was a cardiac cripple, he couldn't get around on his own. He had to sneak smokes. His death wrecked my sister's life. She became a recluse for the next twenty years.

I worked with a person who smoked through the hole in his throat after a laryngectomy from cancer of the throat. (And the tobacco executives testify that nicotine isn't addictive!)

I've seen people with horribly distorted faces due to surgery for mouth cancer.

I lost a sister-in-law to lung cancer at forty-three; another brother-in-law from a sudden heart attack at forty-nine (he was a three-pack-a-day Viceroy smoker); an old friend, cigar smoker, died of kidney cancer after three or four surgeries over ten years; three of my women friends in one year died of lung cancer—all in their early sixties.

I've seen too much suffering, too many premature deaths, and too many bereaved survivors whose lives were unnecessarily wrecked because of cigarettes. Because they were purposely persuaded to smoke when they were children.

If I sound like I have a mission, I must admit, finally, that perhaps I do. I want to do what I can to prevent any unnecessary suffering that tobacco causes.

Now that *you* have quit, I want to ask you to join the fight: Tell people how wonderful you feel now that you don't smoke anymore. Help defuse the myth that it's hard to quit and miserable without cigarettes. Let smokers know how much better you feel now; how much more pep and energy you have, what you're doing with your cigarette money . . . or whatever good happens to you.

If you want to help other smokers quit, I've written a "Facilitator's Guide" that provides directions for leading someone—or a group—through to success using this book. Write to me for information about the guide.

Thank you for your understanding.

P.S.: Don't forget to do the questionnaire on the very last page. I really do want to hear from you.

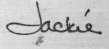

A Word from Those Who Know

Thousands of letters and completed questionnaires from SmokEnder graduates are received each week. Typically, they celebrate the act of quitting and the joy of not-smoking. Smoking is a great equalizer. Quitting is too! Following are a few comments by people who have read the first edition of this book, as well as graduates, which show the diversity in age, occupation and smoking history of SmokEnder members. You can identify with someone who perhaps has smoked as long as you have, or as many packs per day, or has a pressured and demanding position or profession.

Data from the hundreds of thousands of in-depth questionnaires returned by graduates are utilized by universities and others for research in such a way as to preserve the anonymity of our members. The following people have given permission for their names to be used in this book. (The date following each quotation is the date on which the member stopped smoking.)

"I am prouder of having stopped smoking than of almost anything else I have accomplished in the last ten years. I will be forever grateful to SmokEnders."—*Barry Manilow, singer-composer (4/30/76)*

"I can't begin to tell you how much your book has meant to me! I HAVE stopped smoking; an impossible feat until now. I smoked for 25 years and every year I tried to quit right before my birthday; I've always hated the thought of becoming another year older and still a smoker. I can now face my 42nd birthday in March as an ex-smoker. I was so inspired by your book, I feel I can do anything now that I have stopped smoking."—*W. Farmer, Lexington, Kentucky (1/92)*

"Thank you for helping to change my life. I started smoking when I was 14 and continued at 2½ to 3 packs a day for the next 14 years. I couldn't imagine myself without a pack in my pocket or without a cigarette in my hand. I smoked anywhere and everywhere and didn't care if it was legal, what I looked like, who I borrowed from, etc. I smoked through colds and flus. I was miserable.

"So clear and effective and gradual is your program, that I found it easy to follow. I had always thought the only way to quit was 'cold turkey.' But the program in your book really weaned me gently from the addiction and picked apart the habit and the need for cigarettes at certain times and in certain situations.

"Financially, I designated $4 per day to what I call my 'Clean Air Fund.' After 2 years I bought an entire computer system and took a 10 day trip to Mexico. Friends say I'm much happier and calmer. I have gained an incredible amount of self esteem from having quit this way and consider it one of the most important things I have done in my life."—*R. Howard, New York City (11/30/90)*

"Your book has definitely changed my life. I was a 1½-pack-a-day smoker for 20 years. On January 20th, 1989, I stopped smoking. I now have quit for 5 years and will never have another for the rest of my life. I'm totally convinced. In the beginning when I first read your book I was somewhat skeptical. But with every page I read the more convinced I became that smoking was not for me.

"I wanted to quit smoking but didn't know how. Your book showed me how.

"I Thank you.

"My wife thanks you.

"My children thank you.

"My lungs thank you.

"My heart thanks you.

"My whole body thanks you.

"Thank you so very much for showing me the way."
—*G. Zbeetnoff, Orangeville, Ontario*

"Thanks for helping me to stop my destructive 18 year, 1½-pack-a-day smoking habit. I had been feeling a bit desperate about ever quitting for good when I happened across your book. I hemmed and hawed for some weeks, finally set a date to quit, followed your program and quit for good. I have no desire to smoke and am ever grateful I just 'happened' to come across that little book. A $5 investment for a lifetime of improved health—not too bad.

"I work at a newspaper with a number of ex-smokers—who quit on their own. I have empathy for smokers who quit without the benefit of your book, and long for a cigarette."—*L. McNicol, Auburn, New York (3/87)*

". . . I wasn't seriously thinking of 'giving up' but I followed the instruction in your book—just for fun. On the 7th of February 1988 I became an ex-smoker for the first time after ten years of smoking 20 a day. The quality of life has improved so much that I have no intention of 'giving up' non-smoking again. Thank you very much."—*L. Becker, Munich, Germany (2/88)*

". . . The fact that I could keep on smoking did the trick because at that point going without a cigarette would give me a panic attack. I still can't believe it but it worked. This April 12th, 1988, will be one year since I had my last cigarette."—*Mrs. W. Idzuda, Woodbridge, Ontario (4/88)*

"I quit smoking because I was tired of glares from non-smokers in public places, I was tired of going outside in twenty degree weather just to smoke, etc., etc. I read your book and quit smoking on October 24, 1993. A day that I don't think I'll ever forget. Not because it was traumatic or difficult but because it marked the beginning of a new and happier life for me.

"The book provided support and motivation to a person who had resolved to never give up his Camels. I think that in the back of my mind, I really wanted to quit, but I covered it up because I always thought it would be too painful or I didn't have enough willpower.

"Your book showed me things in an entirely different light and taught me things I was very surprised to find out."—*J. Rainwater, Jr., Crownsville, Maryland (10/93)*

"I want to thank you for saving my life. I am a 35-year-old single mother of two girls. My girls have been after me to quit smoking for years. I smoked 2 packs a day for 18 years.

"Now I feel better and people say that I look better and have more energy than I did before I quit smoking. Your book has thrown a light on all those excuses that I used to use to continue smoking. I know I will never smoke again. And the good news is that of all the people I work with, six have quit since they saw that I could do it."—*K. Weikal, Wichita, Kansas (7/87)*

"I still can't believe that after 23 years of smoking that I am free and so pain free.

"The program in your book works perfectly. The habit breaking techniques really made my cut-off day smooth and easy. I had tried all these before, each one alone, to no avail. But combined, they make a powerful statement.

"Wild horses could not make me start on that vicious cycle of a habit again. I WILL live to see more sunsets than ever before possible, thanks to you."—*C. M. Ortega, Walnut, California (2/88)*

"I smoked 2 packs a day for 17 years. I read your book and stopped smoking on February 6, 1988. I'd been trying to quit for the last five years but every time I would go back to smoking. The longest time I went without was for 12 weeks and I felt sorry for myself the whole time. I would sit and wish that I could smoke. It's no wonder I went back every time.

"Your book helped me but I don't know how. I can't really say what is different this time and yet it is. Every morning when I get up I rejoice in my freedom. I AM FREE! And I certainly have no reason to feel sorry for myself. Actually, I feel sorry for others who are still hooked and I pass your book on to smokers I know at every opportunity."—*J. Cantrall, Gilroy, California (2/6/88)*

"Thank you for writing *You CAN Stop Smoking*. I did. Your book is a pure miracle and its effect reaches far beyond the act of quitting the habit. How lucky I am to be free to be myself, thanks to you.

"I've been studying opera for a year and suddenly I'm proud of my ability to sing a high C above middle C.

"I can't thank you enough for the great happiness and fantastic life I have *re-found*! I've even rediscovered not only the courage to believe in myself, but in my dreams. . . ."—*A. Alexander, Dartmouth College (3/91)*

"I think it's a wonderful program. I think it is sensitive and scientific. It's wonderful to feel that someone cares and doesn't condemn your weakness, and at the same time can offer such constructive help, and if the person wants to stop smoking I see no way that it can fail. I offer my heartfelt thanks to God, to SmokEnders and to dear Addie [Addie Gerber, SmokEnders Moderator] for helping me as they have."—*Rosemary Harris, award-winning actress (2/25/76)*

"SmokEnders [quitting smoking] has been the most incredible thing I have ever done for me and me alone. Everything else in a full lifetime had revolved around my husband and children; this is the one thing that has been completely mine."—*Gertrude Eltman, Long Island City, New York, who had smoked between three and four packs a day for almost forty years (7/11/75)*

"I enjoy life more and like myself more."—*J. Messina, Meriden, Connecticut, who had smoked two packs a day for 21 years (2/20/74)*

"I'm now able to run between one and two miles every day—and feel great afterward! Before, ever since I had started to smoke, I couldn't run a hundred yards."—*William Verschuren, Chatham Township, New Jersey, who had smoked two to three packs a day for over fourteen years (2/24/77)*

"I've said it over and over, but I will never stop saying it—thank you so much. I couldn't have done it without you. And not to miss it!! Improvements noticed since quitting: Clean teeth. Great skin color and texture. Hair, too. Altogether much more life."—*Tamara Daniel, actress, New York City (2/22/74)*

"I have truly come to enjoy *not* smoking."—*Melvin Kushner, DDS, Owings Mills, Maryland, who had smoked 1½ packs a day for nineteen years (6/11/76)*

"I have more energy—do not tire as quickly as before while doing anything physical. I feel marvelous. Have no desire to begin smoking again."—*Barbara Goldberg, Flushing, New York, who had smoked 1½ packs a day for 25 years (5/1/74)*

"I feel fantastic. Am I glad I came into contact with SmokEnders at a young age. After previous unsuccessful attempts to quit, SmokEnders was easy."—*John M. Doherty, M.D., Aston, Pa., who had smoked one pack a day for eleven years (3/3/76)*

"SmokEnders is fantastic! It offers a remarkable program to help people quit smoking—calmly, comfortably and permanently. I am personally thankful for SmokEnders. I am thankful for our profession because for the first time we can send the patient who must stop smoking to the one organization that is most likely to help him succeed."—*I. Norton Brotman, DDS, FACD, Clinical Professor of Oral Diagnosis, Dental School, University of Maryland (10/24/75)*

"I have never been happier over stopping something. I feel so much better, I breathe better, my complexion is better, and those cancer commercials no longer bother me."—*Al Malone, St. Petersburg, Florida, who had smoked one pack a day for 42 years (2/26/77)*

"I am more calm and feel better than I have in years. I even have my beverages without thinking of a cigarette. There is no question my self-image has improved, and I am forever grateful to SmokEnders."—*Joan Hillenbrand, Batesville, Indiana, who had smoked 1½ packs a day for 25 years (10/28/76)*

"We can never fully believe we quit smoking so easily. Smoking was something we did continuously. It seemed unlikely that either or both of us could quit. Many thanks."—*Mr. and Mrs. James Durham, Astoria, Oregon (1969)*

"The program provided a number of insights and techniques which I have found valuable in remaining cut off."—*A. R. Hutson, Summit, New Jersey, who had smoked a pack a day for thirty years (2/27/74)*

"Exhilaration is the only word I can think of to adequately describe the feeling of quitting smoking by the SmokEnder method. It's the best life investment I have ever made." —*Ross Reid, Executive Director, Consulting Engineers of Ontario, Toronto, Canada (10/29/76)*

"For the past ten years I have tried various methods (some very expensive) of quitting. Then one day, not long ago, I went through a box of old books and found your book YOU CAN STOP. Well, as suggested, after completing "THE BOOK" I set MY DATE. I ritually smoked my last cigarette . . . put it out—cleaned out and put away all ash trays and I haven't had a puff since!! I'm trying not to gloat over my new freedom, but Jackie, I am so darn proud of myself I can hardly stand it . . . If I find myself having a hard day, I literally say to myself 'but I don't smoke anymore. Life is great—I'm great!' THANK YOU."—*Arlene McKinney, Rescue, California*

"After 25 years of smoking two packs a day, and a number of unsuccessful attempts to stop, I encountered SmokEnders ten years ago, and have been off cigarettes ever since. There have been numerous beneficial effects especially in the health area. I have since looked at the SmokEnder Program from the prospective of a professional who has spent his career studying and treating addiction, and remain impressed by the soundness and ingenuity of the principles upon which it was based. Jackie Rogers has made a major contribution to the health of many Americans and the book, *You Can Stop*, is a lucid exposition of how people can apply what she has developed."—*Herbert D. Kleber, M.D., Professor of Psychiatry, School of Medicine, Yale University (1975), now Director, Division on Substance Abuse, Columbia University College of Physicians and Surgeons.*

Appendices

KARMA STRETCHES
WEEK 1
REPEAT 4 X

1. DEEP BREATHING
A. Stand with feet comfortably apart. Arms at side.
B. Inhale and raise arms overhead. Lower arms as you exhale.

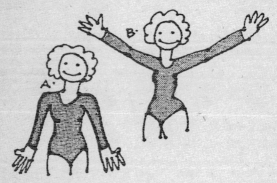

2. SHOULDER ROLLS
(May be done sitting or standing)
A. Stand tall. Back erect. Inhale.
B. Exhale as you roll your shoulder up to your ear, back and down.
C. Repeat on opposite sides. You can do both shoulders together for a change.

3. OVERHEAD REACH

A. Feet hip-width apart. Toes slightly turned out. Knees soft (slightly bent) and abdominals contracted.

B. Raise arms overhead, palms facing each other. Breathe reaching up as though climbing a rope, as you lift clear from the waist up, feeling the ribs move left and right as you stretch. Don't be in a hurry.

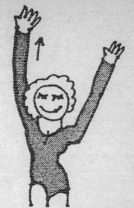

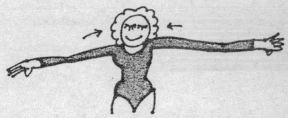

4. SHOULDER SQUEEZE (May be done sitting or standing)

A. Standing tall, feet hip-width apart. Arms out to side.

B. Exhale as you squeeze your shoulder blades together. Inhale, relax, repeat. (This shoulder squeeze can be done throughout the day to relieve tension.)

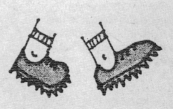

5. RUN IN PLACE for 30 seconds to your favorite beat.

WEEK 2
REPEAT 6 X

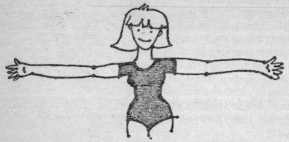

1. ARMS CIRCLE
A. Arms outstretched to sides, palms-out. Feet hip-width apart, toes slightly turned out, knees soft. Shoulders down. Inhale.
B. Exhale and inhale as you rotate six times forward and backward, breathing as you move.

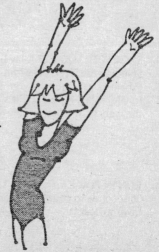

2. SIDE BENDS
A. Stand erect. Inhale as you slowly bring arms upward in line with ears and head.
B. Slowly exhale as you bend and stretch to the right. Inhale coming back to center. Exhale. Tall and tight.

3. **INNER THIGHS STRETCH**
A. Stand tall and tight with feet wide apart. Inhale. Toes out.
B. Exhale as you bend your knees until your hands touch your knees.

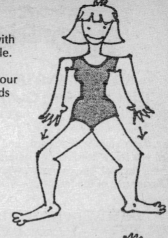

4. **TOE TOUCHES**
A. Stand with feet wide apart, tall and tight.
B. Twist body as you bend over and touch right hand to left foot. Sweep left hand up and back. Return up to center and repeat opposite sides.

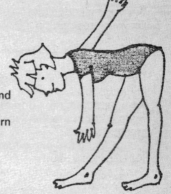

5. **JUMP ROPE OR RUN IN PLACE** for 1 minute to your favorite beat.

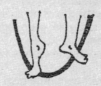

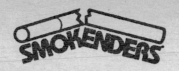

REWARDS AND DISTRACTIONS*
(That Are Neither Costly nor Fattening)

Here's a supply of rewards and distractions to refer to when you feel a desire for a cigarette.

First, decode! Ask yourself "What do I really want?"

Choose one of the following—instead of a cigarette.

DO SOMETHING NICE FOR YOURSELF
YOU DESERVE IT

1. Buy yourself one flower—or pick one just for yourself.
2. Fix your breakfast on a tray and get back into bed and enjoy it.
3. Pack yourself a lunch and picnic in the park during your lunch hour.
4. Fly a kite, play a game of "Frisbee" or buy some liquid bubbles.
5. Try a new cologne, perfume, after-shave.
6. Build a fire in the fireplace, put on some records and create an event.
7. Go for a free makeup demonstration.
8. Join a chorus. Sing!
9. Send a love letter to someone you've been taking for granted.
10. Read an underground newspaper.
11. Have you handwriting analyzed.
12. Write a letter to your legislator and get a gripe off your chest.
13. Call on someone elderly who would really appreciate your visit.
14. Take a twenty-minute nap.
15. Buy a new magazine.
16. Do the relaxation ritual.

17. Take up a new hobby.
18. Take ride into the country . . . smell the clean, fresh air.
19. Get a new hairstyle . . . cut it short, change the color, get a wig. . . .
20. Take a mini-vacation. Overnight in a nearby motel with your mate.
21. Take a bike ride. Feel the breeze blow through your hair.
22. Have a massage.
23. Reserve a bestseller at the library.
24. Respond to a "yours free" ad in a magazine.
25. Adopt a tree on your street and plant some flowers or ivy in its bed.
26. Go roller skating.
27. Rent a rowboat for an hour.
28. Watch birds. Build a birdhouse outside your window.
29. Buy some exotic fresh fruits. Make a wild fruit salad.
30. Browse through a popular, busy health foods store.
31. Go fishing off a public pier. Use bologna for bait.
32. Buy new sneakers!
33. Have a manicure; a pedicure.
34. Buy a lottery ticket.
35. Update your photo album or edit your slide collection.
36. Plant a windowsill herb garden.
37. Adopt a pet from the ASPCA.
38. Turn on some music and dance—by yourself.
39. Read and record for the blind.
40. Have dinner by candlelight.
41. Go for a swim. The "Y" or the club or the old swimming hole.
42. Plan some "me-time."
43. Take a bubble bath or a bracing shower.
44. Sleep late one day this week.
45. Have your teeth cleaned and admire them.
46. Plan a hayride. Be a kid again.
47. Buy yourself some colored felt-tip pens. Draw something.
48. Take calligraphy lessons.
49. Buy a goldfish and care for it.
50. Take up a musical instrument: guitar, recorder, piano, drums. . . .

51. Make paper airplanes and watch them fly.
52. Take a walk through a gentle rain shower or a field of flowers.
53. Take a walk through crunchy autumn leaves.
54. Go to a football game.
55. Romp through the snow. Have a snowball fight with friends.
56. Go skiing or ice skating.
57. Write a letter to an editor. Underscore something positive.
58. Jog before breakfast.
59. Help coach the Little League or the Pop Warner football team.
60. Write a poem about how great you are and how great life is, now that you're free!
61. Watch a spectacular sunrise or a breathtaking sunset.
62. Take art lessons.
63. Raise a sunflower. The biggest one in captivity.
64. Find a secret place to go skinny dipping.
65. Go for a walk in the woods or by the shore. Bring your sketch pad.
66. Have a lemonade during your coffee break.
67. Watch a movie.
68. Solve a crossword puzzle.
69. Make a list of suitable, exciting eating places. Choose one and go.
70. Listen to birdcalls and try to identify them. Buy a bird book.
71. Design your dream house.
72. Play Monopoly with kids and adults in the house.
73. Learn to read faster.
74. Walk in the woods and get to know wildflowers.
75. Research your roots.
76. Sleep out under the stars.
77. Volunteer at party headquarters for the candidate of your choice.
78. Go back to bed after sending the kids off to school.
79. Read your "assets" list and feel cheered.
80. Start writing that book you've been promising you'd write someday.
81. Count the money saved in your money jar!
82. Buy yourself a shirt without a "cigarette pocket."

83. Throw out your ugly ashtrays; turn your nice ones into planters.
84. Exult in self-satisfaction. You DID IT!
85. Clean out your car's ashtray. Use it for tokens, toll money or a small bouquet of artificial flowers.
86. Take your pulse. Now that you quit smoking, it's rewarding to see that it's getting back to normal.
87. Each month, on the anniversary of your Cut-Off, do something wonderful to celebrate.

SYMPTOMS OF RECOVERY: DURATION AND TREATMENT*

NOTE: If a symptom persists or is worrisome, see your doctor

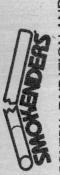

SYMPTOM	AVERAGE DURATION	TREATMENT
DIGESTIVE		
ACID INDIGESTION/HEARTBURN		
The most common digestive problem. The paradox here is smokers who had acid indigestion while they smoked find it disappears; smokers who never had acid indigestion often become troubled with it after they quit.	3 weeks to 3 months. Not the same intensity throughout.	Tums for mild acid indigestion; stronger proprietaries if necessary. Reduction or elimination of acid-producing foods such as caffeine, chocolates and other greasy heartburn-producing items. A suggested remedy; a small cracker to absorb the acid like a blotter—for many, very effective.
NAUSEA		
A very infrequent reaction	1 to 2 weeks. Occasional reports of a day or two of intermittent nausea.	Any usual treatment or just put up with it—it will pass. Suggestion—a teaspoon of Coke Syrup (from the Soda Fountain dispenser).

INCREASED THIRST
Very common

1 to 2 weeks prior to cut-off; several weeks following.

Drink water. Tea, cola, coffee aren't useful for thirst. Your body needs water.

DIARRHEA
Smokers frequently feel they have a virus or the "24 hour bug" after they quit.

Several days in most cases.

Common Sense. Temporarily cut down intake of orange juice and fresh fruits and vegetables.

CONSTIPATION
Rare but of great concern for members who have a history of constipation.

Several weeks to several months.

Use all treatment as prescribed by your physician in the past. Pay special attention to your diet. Avoid cheese, increase fiber. If of long duration, speak to your physician. Nicotine as a drug triggers the bowels in some cases. There are other natural means which can achieve the same results.

GAS (Also called Flatulence)

Generally several weeks at most. However, a few reported cases of extended duration.

Patience. It will soon pass. Temporarily avoid gas-producing food and drinks. Milk can be a cause. If so, Lactaid helps.

(continued)

SYMPTOM	AVERAGE DURATION	TREATMENT
RESPIRATORY		
Generally all gagging coughs, throat clearings, chest tightness and other related respiratory problems disappear very dramatically within the first several weeks. These too are Symptoms of Recovery. The following have been reported as occurring **after** cessation to members who never had these problems before.		
PHLEGM		
This requires constant clearing of the throat and is probably attributable to the awakening of the cilia now that nicotine no longer paralyzes it—a very good sign indeed. It may also be caused by the new natural activity of the nasal passages. Don't be alarmed if you cough up some black phlegm on occasion.	A few days to a few months.	Something hot to drink, gargles, lozenges that cut phlegm, time. Consider avoiding all dairy products. (For some they produce mucus.) Take a calcium supplement.
HOARSENESS		
Similar to above. Many reported cases.	Several weeks to several months.	The same as for phlegm except use soothing lozenges.
SINUS CONGESTION		
This is both a respiratory and a soft tissue condition. A substantial number	A few days to a few months.	Management by physician or self-treatment as indicated.

or graduates have indicated their old sinus conditions erupt for a period of time shortly after Cut-Off.

COUGH

Due to reactivated cilia.	1–2 weeks	Gratitude. The body is restoring itself.

CIRCULATORY

HEIGHTENED AWARENESS AND DIZZINESS

This may be a reaction to the improved circulation and increased oxygen to the brain, now that blood vessels are no longer being constricted by nicotine.	Few days. (Unless caused by low blood pressure.)	Good judgment. Rest. Orange juice. Time to readjust to the normal complement of oxygen in your blood.

LEG PAINS

Improved circulation seems to show itself as cramps in the most commonly affected parts—the legs.	Several weeks.	Elevate the legs, massage, good common sense, time. Increase potassium . . . bananas, orange juice or supplements.

SWELLING/BLOATING

Generally, a result of fluid retention due to decreased caffeine (a diuretic)	Several days to several weeks.	Physician may prescribe mild diuretic. Increased exercise, reduced salt in- (continued)

SYMPTOM	AVERAGE DURATION	TREATMENT
and the counter reaction of nicotine withdrawal which in itself is *not* a diuretic. Swelling may also be caused by changes in the circulatory process—more blood entering extremities which in the past were deprived because of poor circulation.		take, time. Elevate the legs to stimulate the elimination of fluids. Increase foods that are natural diuretics: mushrooms, spinach, asparagus.
STIFFNESS		
See also Leg Pains and Swelling above. Stiffness may be also associated with temporary muscular changes. Relationship of muscular changes to quitting is still little understood.	A few days to a few weeks.	Warm baths. Patience.
TINGLY FINGERS		
Due to improved circulation.	Several weeks.	Patience. It's very good news that the blood is flowing into your extremities again.
MISCELLANEOUS		
DROWSINESS, MUDDLEHEADEDNESS, FATIGUE, SLEEPINESS, LETHARGY.	2–3 weeks	During waking hours, Enerjets, legal snacks especially orange juice, breathing exercise. Cat naps when pos-

INSOMNIA

sible. Physical exercise to stimulate circulation.

Deep breathing. Warm milk and honey before bed. Also, you may require less sleep due to quitting. Many people can function beautifully on 4 or 5 hours sleep.

BLEEDING GUMS

Very common. It's a paradox that bleeding occurs as a result of quitting.

4–8 weeks

Amosan Mouthwash. If condition persists, prompt treatment by a dentist is required. If your dentist would like an explanation of this phenomenon, show or give him the "Bleeding Gums" letter in the Appendices section.

IRRITABILITY

If due to fluid retention, refer to Circulatory Section under Swelling, for suggested treatment. Also, may be labeled "irritability" by others when it is truly "independence." In time, the need to assert oneself normalizes.

(continued)

SYMPTOM	TREATMENT
ALSO: ITCHINESS NERVOUSNESS SHOOTING PAINS EXCITEMENT (Euphoria) DEPRESSION VISION CHANGES SALT HUNGER EXCESSIVE SALIVATION METALLIC TASTE RESIDUAL TOBACCO TASTE SORE TONGUE LOW ALCOHOL THRESHOLD HEADACHE THYROID CHANGES	Blame everything bad on smoking; everything good on quitting. Remember each symptom is evidence that your body is repairing itself.

BLEEDING GUMS LETTER

From the desk of Jon Rogers, DDS

Dear Doctor,

Your patient has recently stopped smoking with the help of our book, *You Can Stop Smoking*, the Smok-Ender method.

Congratulations are in order.

However, your patient is now concerned about a common oral condition following cessation: "bleeding gums."

Permit me to shed some light on this. As co-founder of SmokEnders, in 1969, I have had the privilege of studying data collected on many thousands of smokers who have gone through the SmokEnder program. This has given me insights into the unique oral physiology/pathology concomitant with smoking cessation. The paradox of gingival problems as a *result* of cessation is little known.

Typically, smokers average 1½ packs of cigarettes a day and have smoked perhaps from ten to twenty-plus years. Consider, then, that during that time, the oral tissues have been subjected to abnormal heat, the products of combustion, nicotine, CO and CO_2, hydrocarbons, residual plant pesticides, etc.

In order to maintain homeostasis, it is reasonable to expect that the soft tissues react to the above insults, and create an excessive layer of surface cornification and atrophy of the exquisite superficial cutaneous nerve endings. A "masking" effect.

As a result, upon cessation, when irritants are removed and the "coating" dissipates, the denuded tissues are tender and more easily subject to irritation during this transitional period. With such drastic change in the environment, there may also be marked changes in oral flora.

During the smoking years the constant exposure of the superficial small blood vessels to the *vasoconstricting* action of nicotine may create a "dependency" upon the nicotine to maintain the patency of these vessel walls.

We believe that upon cessation, the abrupt discontinuation of this vasoconstrictor to the small vessels and capillaries of the oral mucous membranes results in transitional flaccidity of the capillary walls and frank unprovoked gingival hemorrhage. The usual period of time for the tissue to regain normal physiology is four to eight weeks.

Additionally, the sloughing off of the cornified layer leaves the normal gingival tissues "unprotected" and more easily irritated. The presence of calcific material, which in itself would have caused gingival bleeding—except for the constant dosing of the vasoconstrictor, nicotine—must be attended.

In my practice, a thorough curettage and prophylaxis together with an increase of vitamin C to 1000 mg per day usually obtain good results.

Any such "symptoms of recovery" which persist beyond this time are usually symptoms of a periodontal condition being "unmasked," and the patient should be promptly treated or referred to the appropriate specialty. Hopefully, the patient will have stopped smoking before too much damage was done.

Inasmuch as your patient has expressed concern to us, I hope the foregoing has shed some light on the subject.

Sincerely,

JON ROGERS, DDS

NICOTINE RATING CHART

NICOTINE CONTENT PER CIGARETTE
From Federal Trade Commission
as of 1993

United States brands do not list nicotine content on packages. For information about nicotine levels of U.S. brands not listed, or for ratings after 1993, call FTC Special Services 202-326-2222.

Canadian brands list nicotine rating on the packs.

Check this list carefully to be sure you are not exceeding the nicotine level required each week. It's important that you don't guess. Be sure you choose the exact brand/style at the correct level. This is a partial list. If the brand you want isn't on this list, call the FTC.

CODE: F=Filter, NF=Non-Filter, MEN=Menthol, HP =Hard Pack, SP=Soft Pack, REG=Regular (70mm), K=King Size (80-85mm), 100 & 120 mm, LT=Light, FLA=Flavor, UL=Ultra Light

NIC: Total alkaloids reported as milligrams of nicotine per cigarette.

BRAND NAME	DESCRIPTION	NIC
ALPINE	KING F SP MEN	1.0
ALPINE	100 F SP MEN	1.1
ALPINE	KING F SP MEN LT	0.7
ALPINE	100 F SP MEN LT	0.7
ALPINE	80 F HP MEN FUL FLA	1.0
ALPINE	80 F HP MEN L	0.7
AMERICAN FILTER	100 F SP	1.3
AMERICAN FILTER	KING F SP	1.3
AMERICAN LIGHTS	100 F SP LT	1.0
AMERICAN LIGHTS	KING F SP LT	0.9
AMERICAN LIGHTS	100 F SP MEN LT	0.9
B & H DE-NIC	KING F HP MEN LT	0.1
B & H DE-NIC	100 F HP LT	0.1
B & H DE-NIC	100 F HP MEN LT	0.1
B & H DE-NIC	KING F HP LT	0.1
BARCLAY	KING F HP	0.3
BARCLAY	KING F SP	0.3
BARCLAY	100 F SP	0.4
BASIC	KING F SP	1.1

BRAND NAME	DESCRIPTION	NIC
BASIC	100 F SP	1.2
BASIC	KING F SP LT	0.8
BASIC	KING F SP MEN LT	0.8
BASIC	100 F SP LT	0.8
BASIC	100 F SP MEN LT	0.8
BASIC	KING F SP ULTRA LT	0.5
BASIC	100 F SP ULTRA LT	0.5
BASIC	KING NF SP	1.6
BELAIR	KING F SP MEN	0.8
BELAIR	100 F SP MEN	0.8
BELAIR	KING F SP MEN LO PRICE	1.2
BELAIR	100 F SP MEN LO PRICE	1.2
BELAIR	KING F SP MEN LT LO PRICE	0.8
BELAIR	100 F SP MEN LT LO PRICE	0.9
BENSON AND HEDGES	KING F HP	1.2
BENSON AND HEDGES	100 F HP LT	0.8
BENSON AND HEDGES	100 F HP MEN LT	0.8
BENSON AND HEDGES	100 F SP	1.1
BENSON AND HEDGES	100 F HP	1.1
BENSON AND HEDGES	100 F HP MEN	1.1
BENSON AND HEDGES	100 F SP MEN	1.1
BENSON AND HEDGES	100 F SP LT	0.8
BENSON AND HEDGES	100 F SP MEN LT	0.8
BENSON AND HEDGES	100 F HP DLX ULTRA LT	0.5
BENSON AND HEDGES	100 F HP MEN DLX ULTRA LT	0.4
BENSON AND HEDGES	KING F SP MULTI	0.9
BEST BUY	KING F SP FUL FLA	1.1
BEST BUY	100 F SP FUL FLA	1.2
BEST BUY	KING F SP LT	0.8
BEST BUY	KING F SP MEN LT	0.8
BEST BUY	100 F SP LT	0.8
BEST BUY	100 F SP MEN LT	0.8
BEST BUY	KING F SP ULTRA LT	0.5
BEST BUY	100 F SP ULTRA LT	0.5
BEST BUY	KING NF SP	1.6
BEST VALUE	KING F SP FUL FLA	1.2
BEST VALUE	100 F SP FUL FLA	1.2
BEST VALUE	KING F SP LT	0.9
BEST VALUE	100 F SP LT	0.8
BEST VALUE	100 F SP ULTRA LT	0.5
BEST VALUE	KING F SP MEN LT	0.9
BEST VALUE	100 F SP MEN LT	1.0
BEST VALUE	KING F SP ULTRA LT	0.5
BIG MONEY	100 F SP MEN LT	0.8
BRISTOL	KING F SP LT	0.8
BRISTOL	KING F SP MEN LT	0.8

BRAND NAME	DESCRIPTION	NIC
BRISTOL	100 F SP LT	0.8
BRISTOL	100 F SP MEN LT	0.9
BRISTOL	KING F SP	1.1
BRISTOL	100 F SP	1.1
BRISTOL	KING NF SP	1.7
BRISTOL	100 F SP ULTRA LT	0.6
BRISTOL	KING F SP LOWEST	0.1
BRISTOL	100 F SP LOWEST	0.2
BUCKS	KING F SP	1.0
BUCKS	KING F SP LT	0.7
BULL DURHAM	KING F HP	1.1
BULL DURHAM	KING F HP LT	0.8
CAMBRIDGE	100 F SP ULTRA	0.4
CAMBRIDGE	KING F SP LT	0.8
CAMBRIDGE	KING F SP MEN LT	0.9
CAMBRIDGE	100 F SP LT	0.8
CAMBRIDGE	100 F SP MEN LT	0.8
CAMBRIDGE	KING F SP FUL FLA	1.1
CAMBRIDGE	100 F SP FUL FLA	1.1
CAMBRIDGE	KING F SP LOWEST	0.1
CAMBRIDGE	100 F SP LOWEST	0.2
CAMEL	KING F SP	1.1
CAMEL	KING F HP	1.2
CAMEL	100 F SP LT	0.8
CAMEL	KING F SP LT	0.8
CAMEL	KING F HP LT	0.7
CAMEL	70 NF SP	1.5
CAMEL	100 F SP	1.1
CAMEL	85 F SP ULTRA LT	0.6
CAMEL	85 F HP ULTRA LT	0.5
CAMEL	100 F HP ULTRA LT	0.6
CAMEL	99 F HP	1.3
CAMEL	98 F HP LT	0.7
CAPRI	100 F HP	0.8
CAPRI	100 F HP MEN	0.7
CAPRI	120 F HP	1.0
CAPRI	120 F HP MEN	0.9
CARLTON	120 F SP	0.5
CARLTON	KING F SP	0.1
CARLTON	120 F SP MEN	0.5
CARLTON	KING F SP MEN	0.1
CARLTON	KING F HP	0.2
CARLTON	100 F HP	0.1
CARLTON	100 F SP	0.2
CARLTON	100 F HP MEN	0.1
CARLTON	100 F SP MEN	0.2

BRAND NAME	DESCRIPTION	NIC
CARLTON	KING F HP ULTRA	<0.05
CARTIER VENDOME	100 F HP	0.7
CARTIER VENDOME	100 F HP 100	0.7
CARTIER VENDOME	100 F HP MEN	0.7
CARTIER VENDOME	100 F HP MEN 10	0.7
CHESTERFIELD	REG NF SP	1.1
CHESTERFIELD	KING NF SP	1.4
CHESTERFIELD	KING F SP LT	0.7
CHESTERFIELD	100 F SP LT	0.8
DORAL	KING F SP LT	0.8
DORAL	KING F SP MEN LT	0.9
DORAL	100 F SP LT	0.9
DORAL	100 F SP MEN LT	0.7
DORAL	KING F SP FUL FLA	1.2
DORAL	100 F SP FUL FLA	1.2
DORAL	100 F SP ULTRA LT	0.5
DORAL	KING F SP MEN FUL FLA	1.2
DORAL	100 F SP MEN FUL FLA	1.2
DORAL	KING F SP ULTRA LT	0.5
ENGLISH OVAL	KING NF HP	1.9
EVE	120 F HP LT	1.0
EVE	120 F HP MEN LT	1.0
EVE	120 F HP ULTRA LT	0.5
EVE	120 F HP MEN ULTRA LT	0.5
EVE	100 F HP MEN ULTRA LT SLIM	0.6
EVE	100 F HP ULTRA LT SLIM	0.5
GENERIC	KING F SP ULTRA LT	0.7
GENERIC	100 F SP ULTRA LT	0.7
GENERIC	KING F SP MEN LT	1.0
GENERIC	KING F SP LT	1.0
GENERIC	100 F SP MEN LT	1.1
GENERIC	100 F SP LT	1.1
GENERIC	KING F HP LT	1.0
GOLDEN LIGHTS	KING F SP LT	0.7
GOLDEN LIGHTS	KING F SP MEN LT	0.7
GOLDEN LIGHTS	100 F SP LT	0.8
GOLDEN LIGHTS	100 F SP MEN LT	0.8
GOLDEN LIGHTS	KING F HP LT	0.6
GOLDEN LIGHTS	100 F HP LT	0.7
HARLEY DAVIDSON	KING F SP	0.8
HARLEY DAVIDSON	KING F SP LT	0.7
HERBERT TAREYTON	KING NF SP	1.7
HERITAGE LIGHTS	100 F SP LT	0.9
HERITAGE LIGHTS	KING F SP LT	0.9
HI-LITE	100 F HP	1.1
KENT	KING F SP	0.9

BRAND NAME	DESCRIPTION	NIC
KENT	100 F SP	0.9
KENT	KING F HP	0.8
KENT	100 F SP MEN	1.0
KENT	KING F SP III	0.4
KENT	100 F SP PLAIN III	0.5
KENT	100 F HP III	0.4
KOOL	100 F SP MEN SUPER LG	1.2
KOOL	REG NF SP MEN	1.3
KOOL	KING F SP MEN	1.1
KOOL	KING F HP MEN	1.0
KOOL	KING F SP MEN LT	0.7
KOOL	100 F SP MEN LT	0.7
KOOL	KING F SP MEN MILD	0.9
KOOL	100 F SP MEN MILD	0.9
KOOL	KING F SP MEN ULTRA	0.2
KOOL	100 F SP MEN ULTRA	0.5
KOOL	KING F HP MEN MILD	0.9
KOOL	KING F SP MEN ULTRA LT	0.6
KOOL	LONG F SP MEN ULTRA LT	0.6
KOOL DELUXE	KING F HP MEN LT	0.8
KOOL DELUXE	LONG F HP MEN LT	0.9
KOOL DELUXE	LONG F HP MEN ULTRA LONG	0.6
L AND M	KING F SP	1.0
L AND M	KING F HP	0.9
L AND M	100 F SP LT 30	0.9
L AND M	100 F SP LT LONG	0.8
L AND M	100 F SP SUPER KING	0.9
L AND M	100 F SP FUL 10PK-30	1.1
L AND M	100 F SP ULT LT 10PK-30	0.5
LARK	KING F SP LT	0.9
LARK	100 F SP LT	1.0
LARK	KING F SP	1.0
LARK	100 F SP EXTRA LONG	1.1
LUCKY STRIKE	REG NF SP	1.6
LUCKY STRIKE	KING F SP	1.0
LUCKY STRIKE	KING F HP	1.0
LUCKY STRIKE	100 F SP	1.1
LUCKY STRIKE	KING F SP LT	0.7
LUCKY STRIKE	100 F SP LT	0.8
MAGNA	KING F SP	1.2
MAGNA	KING F HP	1.2
MAGNA	KING F SP LT	0.8
MAGNA	KING F HP LT	0.8
MALIBU	100 F SP	1.2
MALIBU	100 F SP LT	0.8
MALIBU	100 F SP MEN	1.0

BRAND NAME	DESCRIPTION	NIC
MALIBU	KING F SP	1.2
MALIBU	KING F SP LT	0.7
MALIBU	KING F SP MEN	1.3
MALIBU	100 F SP ULTRA LT	0.5
MARLBORO	79 F HP	1.1
MARLBORO	KING F SP	1.1
MARLBORO	KING F SP 25	1.1
MARLBORO	KING F SP MEN	1.0
MARLBORO	100 F SP	1.2
MARLBORO	100 F HP	1.1
MARLBORO	KING F SP LT	0.8
MARLBORO	KING F SP LT 25	0.8
MARLBORO	KING F HP LT	0.8
MARLBORO	100 F SP LT	0.8
MARLBORO	100 F HP LT	0.8
MARLBORO	100 F P MEN LT	0.8
MARLBORO	KING F HP MEN LT	0.8
MARLBORO	KING F HP ULTRA LT	0.5
MARLBORO	100 F HP ULTRA LT	0.5
MARLBORO	KING F HP MEN	1.0
MARLBORO	KING F HP MEDIUM	0.8
MARLBORO	KING F SP MEDIUM	0.8
MAX	120 F SP	1.2
MAX	120 F SP MEN	1.2
MERIT	KING F SP	0.6
MERIT	KING F SP MEN	0.6
MERIT	100 F SP	0.8
MERIT	100 F SP MEN	0.8
MERIT	KING F HP	0.6
MERIT	KING F SP ULTRA LT	0.5
MERIT	100 F SP ULTRA LT	0.5
MERIT	KING F SP MEN ULTRA LT	0.4
MERIT	100 F SP MEN ULTRA LT	0.5
MERIT	KING F HP ULTRA LT	0.4
MERIT	100 F HP ULTRA LT	0.5
MERIT DE-NIC	KING F SP	0.1
MERIT DE-NIC	KING F SP MEN	0.1
MERIT DE-NIC	KING F SP ULTRA	0.1
MERIT DE-NIC	KING F SP MEN ULTRA	0.1
MONTCLAIR	100 F SP	1.2
MONTCLAIR	100 F SP LT	1.0
MONTCLAIR	100 F SP MEN LT	1.0
MONTCLAIR	KING F SP LT	0.9
MONTCLAIR	KING F SP MEN LT	0.9
MONTCLAIR	KING F SP	1.2
MONTCLAIR	100 F SP ULTRA LT	0.5

BRAND NAME	DESCRIPTION	NIC
MORE	120 F SP	1.2
MORE	100 F HP LT	0.8
MORE	120 F SP MEN	1.4
MORE	100 F HP MEN LT	0.7
MORE	120 F SP MEN LT	1.0
MORE	120 F SP LT	0.9
MORE	120 F SP WHT LT	0.9
MORE	120 F SP MEN WHT LT	1.0
NEWPORT	KING F SP MEN	1.3
NEWPORT	KING F SP MEN 25	1.3
NEWPORT	100 F SP MEN	1.4
NEWPORT	100 F SP MEN 25	1.4
NEWPORT	KING F HP MEN	1.2
NEWPORT	KING F SP MEN LT	0.7
NEWPORT	100 F SP MEN LT	0.8
NEWPORT	KING F HP MEN LT	0.8
NEWPORT	100 F HP MEN	1.4
NEWPORT	100 F HP MEN LT	0.7
NEWPORT	100 F HP STRIPES	0.9
NEWPORT STRIPE	100 F HP MEN SLIM LT	0.8
NEWPORT STRIPE	100 F HP	0.9
NEXT	KING F SP MEN LO TAR	0.1
NEXT	100 F SP LO TAR	0.1
NEXT*	100 F SP MEN LO TAR	0.1
NEXT*	KING F SP ULTRA LO TAR	0.1
NEXT*	KING F SP MEN ULTRA LO TAR	0.1
NEXT*	100 F SP ULTRA LO TAR	0.1
NEXT*	100 F SP MEN ULTRA LO TAR	0.1
NEXT	KING F SP LO TAR	0.1
NO FRILLS	KING F SP LT	0.8
NO FRILLS	KING F SP MEN LT	0.8
NO FRILLS	100 F SP LT	0.8
NO FRILLS	100 F SP ULTRA LT	0.5
NO FRILLS	100 F SP FUL FLA	1.2
NO FRILLS	100 F SP MEN LT	0.8
NO FRILLS	KING F SP ULTRA LT	0.5
NO FRILLS	KING F SP	1.1
NOW	100 F SP	0.2
NOW	KING F SP	0.1
NOW	100 F SP MEN	0.2
NOW	KING F SP MEN	0.1
NOW	KING F HP	<0.05
NOW	100 F HP	<0.05
OLD GOLD	KING F SP	1.3
OLD GOLD	100 F SP	1.4
OLD GOLD	KING NF SP STRIGHT	1.8

BRAND NAME	DESCRIPTION	NIC
OLD GOLD	KING F SP LT	0.7
OLD GOLD	100 F SP LT	1.0
PALL MALL	KING NF SP	1.8
PALL MALL	100 F SP LT	0.8
PALL MALL	100 F SP	1.2
PALL MALL	KING F SP RED	1.2
PALL MALL	100 F SP RED	1.2
PALL MALL	100 F SP LT	1.2
PARLIAMENT	KING F HP LT	0.7
PARLIAMENT	KING F SP LT	0.7
PARLIAMENT	100 F SP LT	0.9
PHILIP MORRIS	KING NF SP COM	1.7
PHILIP MORRIS	REG NF SP	1.4
PHILIP MORRIS	100 F HP INTL	1.1
PHILIP MORRIS	100 F HP MEN INTL	1.2
PICAYUNE	REG NF SP	1.2
PLAYERS	REG NF HP	1.8
PLAYERS	KING F HP	0.8
PLAYERS	KING F HP MEN	0.8
PLAYERS	100 F HP	1.0
PLAYERS	100 F HP MEN	1.0
PLAYERS	KING F SP LT 25	0.8
PLAYERS	KING F SP MEN LT 25	0.8
PLAYERS	100 F SP LT 25	0.9
PLAYERS	100 F SP MEN LT 25	0.9
PYRAMID	KING F SP LT	0.8
PYRAMID	100 F SP LT	0.9
PYRAMID	100 F SP MEN LT	0.9
PYRAMID	KING NF SP	1.3
PYRAMID	100 F SP ULTRA LT	0.5
PYRAMID	KING F SP FUL FLA	1.0
PYRAMID	KING F SP MEN FUL FLA	1.0
PYRAMID	100 F SP FUL FLA	1.1
PYRAMID	100 F SP MEN FUL FLA	1.1
RALEIGH	KING F SP	1.0
RALEIGH	100 F SP	1.0
RALEIGH	KING F SP LT	0.9
RALEIGH	100 F SP LT	0.9
RALEIGH	REG NF SP	1.4
RICHLAND	KING F SP	1.2
RICHLAND	KING F SP 25	1.2
RICHLAND	KING F SP MEN	1.1
RICHLAND	KING F SP MEN 25	1.0
RICHLAND	KING F SP LT 25	0.9
RICHLAND	KING F SP LT	0.9
RICHLAND	100 F SP	1.3

BRAND NAME	DESCRIPTION	NIC
RICHLAND	100 F SP 25	1.3
RICHLAND	100 F SP LT	1.0
RICHLAND	100 F SP LT 25	0.9
RICHLAND	100 F SP MEN LONG	1.1
RITZ	100 F HP MEN	0.9
RITZ	100 F HP	0.8
SALEM	KING F SP MEN	1.3
SALEM	85 F HP MEN	1.2
SALEM	100 F SP MEN LT	0.7
SALEM	KING F SP MEN LT	0.7
SALEM	100 F SP MEN	1.2
SALEM	100 F HP MEN SLIM LT	0.7
SALEM	KING F SP MEN ULTRA LT	0.4
SALEM	100 F SP MEN ULTRA LT	0.4
SARATOGA	120 F HP	1.1
SARATOGA	120 F HP MEN	1.1
SATIN	100 F SP	0.9
SATIN	100 F SP MEN	0.9
SAVVY	100 F SP LT	0.9
SAVVY	100 F SP MEN LT	0.9
SAVVY	100 F SP ULTRA LT	0.5
SCOTCH BUY	KING F SP FUL FLA	1.2
SCOTCH BUY	100 F SP FUL FLA	1.2
SCOTCH BUY	KING F SP LT	0.9
SCOTCH BUY	100 F SP LT 100	0.8
SCOTCH BUY	KING F SP MEN LT	0.9
SCOTCH BUY	100 F SP MEN LT	1.0
SCOTCH BUY	100 F SP ULTRA LT	0.5
SCOTCH BUY	KING F SP ULTRA LT	0.5
SILVA THINS	100 F HP	0.9
SILVA THINS	100 F HP MEN	1.0
SPRING	100 F SP MEN	1.5
SPRING	KING F SP MEN LEMON LT	0.7
SPRING	100 F SP MEN LT LEMON	0.8
STERLING	100 F SP FUL FLA	1.1
STERLING	100 F SP MEN FUL FLA	1.2
STERLING	100 F SP LT	0.8
STERLING	100 F SP MEN LT	0.8
STERLING	KING F SP FUL FLA	1.0
STERLING	KING F SP MEN FUL FLA	1.0
STERLING	KING F SP LT	0.8
STERLING	KING F SP MEN LT	0.7
STERLING	100 F HP SLIM LT	0.7
STERLING	100 F HP MEN SLIM LT	0.7
STERLING	100 F SP ULTRA LT	0.4
STERLING	100 F SP MEN ULTRA LT	0.4

BRAND NAME	DESCRIPTION	NIC
TAREYTON	KING F SP	1.0
TAREYTON	100 F SP	1.0
TAREYTON	KING F SP LT	0.5
TAREYTON	100 F SP LONG LT	0.7
TRIUMPH	KING F SP	0.3
TRIUMPH	KING F SP MEN	0.4
TRIUMPH	100 F SP	0.4
TRIUMPH	100 F SP MEN	0.5
TRUE	KING F SP	0.4
TRUE	KING F SP MEN	0.4
TRUE	100 F SP	0.6
TRUE	100 F SP MEN	0.6
TRUE	KING F HP	0.4
TRUE	100 F HP	0.6
VANTAGE	100 F SP	0.7
VANTAGE	KING F SP	0.6
VANTAGE	100 F SP ULTRA LT	0.4
VANTAGE	KING F SP ULTRA LT	0.4
VANTAGE	KING F SP MEN	0.7
VANTAGE	100 F SP MEN	0.6
VICEROY	KING F SP	1.2
VICEROY	100 F SP	1.2
VICEROY	KING F SP LT	0.9
VICEROY	100 F SP LT	0.9
VICEROY	KING F HP	1.1
VICEROY	100 F HP	1.2
VICEROY	KING F HP LT	0.9
VICEROY	100 F HP LT	0.9
VIRGINIA SLIMS	100 F SP SLIM	1.0
VIRGINIA SLIMS	100 F SP MEN SLIM	1.0
VIRGINIA SLIMS	100 F HP SLIM LT	0.7
VIRGINIA SLIMS	100 F HP MEN SLIM LT	0.7
VIRGINIA SLIMS	100 F HP ULTRA LT	0.5
WINSTON	100 F SP	1.1
WINSTON	KING F SP	1.5
WINSTON	KING F HP	1.2
WINSTON	100 F SP LT	0.8
WINSTON	KING F SP LT	0.7
WINSTON	KING F HP LT	0.7
WINSTON	100 F SP ULTRA LT	0.4
WINSTON	KING F SP ULTRA LT	0.6
WINSTON	100 F HP LT	0.8

IN CANADA:
Nicotine Values by rank.

Camel, K,F	1.6	Sweet Cap Plain, R	1.3
More 120,	1.6	Sweet Cap, R,F	1.3
More Menthol 120	1.6	Zel,	1.3
Winston 100, F	1.6	Gauloise Uni, R	1.25
Peter Jackson, K,F	1.5	Avanti 100	1.2
Players, K,F	1.5	Avant, K,F	1.2
Sweet Cap, K,F	1.5	B & H 100, F	1.2
Winston, F,R	1.5	B & H 100 Menthol	1.2
Belvedere, K	1.4	B & H Special, K,F	1.2
Black Cat, K,F	1.4	B & H Special Light, K,F	1.2
Camel, R,NF	1.4	Belvedere Extra Mild, K	1.2
Cameo Menthol, K,F	1.4	Belvedere Light, R	1.2
Export, R,F	1.4	Black Cat Light, K,F	1.2
Gitane Uni, NF,R	1.4	Carven A, K,F	1.2
Mark Ten Plain, K	1.4	Du Maurier, R,F	1.2
Pall Mall, F,K	1.4	Export A Medium, K	1.2
Players Medium, K,F	1.4	Export A Medium, R,F	1.2
Players, R,F	1.4	Mark Ten, K	1.2
Players Special Blend, K,F	1.4	Mark Ten, K,F	1.2
Players Special Blend, R,F	1.4	Number 7, K,F	1.2
Salem, K,F	1.4	Number 7 Light, R,F	1.2
Salem Light, K,F	1.4	Peter Stuyvesant, R,F	1.2
Du Maurier, K,F	1.3	Peter Stuyvesant, 100, F	1.2
Dunhill, K,F	1.3	Rothman's, K,F	1.2
Export A,K	1.3	Sportsman, K,F	1.2
Export A, R,F	1.3	Winston Light 100, F	1.2
Macdonald Special, K,F	1.3	Belvedere Extra Mild, R	1.1
Macdonald Special, R,F	1.3	Cameo, K,F	1.1
Mark Ten Light, R,F	1.3	Craven Menthol, K,F	1.1
Mark Ten, R,F	1.3	Du Maurier Light, K,F	1.1
No Name Virginia	1.3	Du Maurier Light, R,F	1.1
No Name Virginia, K,F	1.3	Du Maurier Special 100, F	1.1
Number 7, R,F	1.3	Du Maurier Special Mild	1.1
Players Light, K,F	1.3	Export A Mild, K	1.1
Players Light, R,F	1.3	Export A Mild, R,F	1.1
Players Medium, R,F	1.3	Kool Menthol Mild, K,F	1.1
Players Plain, R	1.3	Macdonald Menthol, K,F	1.1
Sergaz, K,F	1.3	Macdonald Special	
Sportsman Plain, R	1.3	Light, K,F	1.1

Brand	Value
Macdonald Special Light, R,F	1.1
Mark Ten Light, K,F	1.1
Matinee, K,F	1.1
Number 7 Light, K,F	1.1
Players Extra Light, K,F	1.1
Rothmans Extra Light, K,F	1.1
Rothmans Light, K,F	1.1
Rothmans Special Mild, K,F	1.1
Vantage 100, R,F	1.1
B & H 100, Light, F	1.0
B & H 100 Light Menthol, F	1.0
Craven A Light, K,F	1.0
Du Maurier Extra Light, K,F	1.0
Du Maurier Special, K,F	1.0
Export A Extra Light, K,F	1.0
Export A Light, K	1.0
Macdonald Menthol, R,F	1.0
Macdonald Special Ex Light, K,F	1.0
Matinee Special 100, K,F	1.0
Matinee Special Mild 100, F	1.0
Matinee Special Mild, K,F	1.0
Matinee Special Mild Menthol, K	1.0
No Name Virginia Light, K,F	1.0
Peter Jackson Light, K,F	1.0
Players Extra Light, R,F	1.0
Rothmans Special Mild 100, F	1.0
Salem 100 Light, F	1.0
Vantage, K,F	1.0
Winston Light, K,F	1.0
Gauloise Blondes, R,F	0.99
Gauloise Filtre, R,F	0.94
Avanti Light 100	0.9
Belmont Mild, K	0.9
Camel Light, K,F	0.9
Cameo Extra Mild Menthol, K,F	0.9
Cameo Special 100, F	0.9
Contessa Slims, K,F	0.9
Craven A, R,F	0.9
Craven A Special Mild 100, F	0.9
Craven A Superslims, F	0.9
Craven Special Mild 100, F,M	0.9
Craven Special Mild 100, F	0.9
Du Maurier Extra Light, R,F	0.9
Export A, Extra Light, R	0.9
Export A, Ultra, Light, K,F	0.9
Macdonald Menthol Light, R,F	0.9
Macdonald Special Ex Light, R,F	0.9
Matinee, R,F	0.9
Matinee Special, K,F	0.9
Salem Light, R,F	0.9
Gitanes, R,F	0.89
Gitanes Legeres, R,F	0.81
Avanti Light, K,F	0.8
B & H 100 Deluxe Ultra Lt, F	0.8
B & H 100 Deluxe Ultra Lt, F,M	0.8
Export A Ultra Lt, R,F	0.8
Craven A Light, R,F	0.7
Belvedere, R,F	0.5
Craven A Special Mild, R,F	0.5
Macdonald Sel Spec Mild, K,F,M	0.5
Macdonald Sel Spec Mild, K,F	0.5
Vantage Light, K,F	0.5
Vantage Light Special, K	0.5
Vantage Menthol Light, K,F	0.5
Viscount Extra Mild, R,F	0.5
Craven A Special Mild, K,F	0.4

Craven Menthol Special Mild, K,F	0.4
Matinee Extra Mild, K,F	0.4
Matinee Extra Mild, R,F	0.4
Matinee Slims Extra Mild, K,F	0.4
Matinee Slims Extra Mild, K,M	0.4
Matinee Slims 100 Ex Mild, F,M	0.4
Peter Jackson Extra Light, K,F	0.4
Viscount 100 Extra Mild, K,	0.4
Viscount Extra Mild, K,F	0.4
Viscount Extra Mild, K,F,M	0.4
Accord Ultra Mild, K	0.3
Accord Ultra Mild Menthol	0.3
Macdonald Select Ultra Mild, K	0.2
Medallion Ultra Mild, K,F	0.2
Craven A Ultra Mild, K,F	0.1
Viscount 1, Ultra Mild, K,F	0.09
Matinee Slims 100 Ex Mild, F	0.05

COST OF SMOKING CHART

Calculate the amount you spend on cigarettes, by the week, month and year. Use the dollar amount closest to the current price per pack. (If cigarettes cost more than $5—say $7 per pack—add the amounts from the $4 and the $3 column.) Transfer the annual amount your spend to the worksheet, item 4. (If more than one person smokes in the household, calculate on the basis of total number of packs per day smoked in that household, as well.) This will give you graphic proof of the money you spend on smoking—and the amount you will save when you quit.

This is the amount you will put into your Cigarette Money savings jar every *night*, after you quit. Plan wonderful rewards for yourself: three weeks after quitting, then three months, and one year.

Study the following compound interest charts to calculate how your "newfound" money will accumulate. It's astounding! What an easy way to make a fortune.

PACKS PER DAY	$2 PER PACK			$2.50 PER PACK			$3.00 PER PACK			$4.00 PER PACK			$5.00 PER PACK		
	PER WEEK	PER MONTH	PER YEAR	PER WEEK	PER MONTH	PER YEAR	PER WEEK	PER MONTH	PER YEAR	PER WEEK	PER MONTH	PER YEAR	PER WEEK	PER MONTH	PER YEAR
1	$14.	$60.	$720.	$17.	$72.	$903.	$21.	$90.	$1083.	$28.	$120.	$1444.	$35.	$150.	$1806.
1½	21.	95.	1140.	26.	112.	1354.	31.	135.	1625.	33.	142.	1702.	52.	226.	2709.
2	28.	120.	1440.	35.	145.	1806.	42.	180.	2160.	56.	240.	2889.	70.	301.	3612.
2½	35.	150.	1800.	43.	188.	2287.	52.	225.	2709.	70.	301.	3612.	87.	376.	4515.
3	42.	180.	2160.	52.	228.	2709.	63.	270.	3250.	84.	361.	4334.	105.	451.	5418.
3½	49.	210.	2520.	61.	263.	3160.	73.	316.	3792.	98.	421.	5057.	122.	526.	6321.
4	56.	240.	2880.	70.	301.	3612.	84.	361.	4334.	112.	482.	5779.	140.	602.	7224.
4½	63.	270.	3240.	78.	338.	4063.	94.	406.	4876.	126.	542.	6502.	157.	667.	8127.
5	70.	300.	3600.	82.	376.	4515.	105.	451.	5418.	140.	602.	7224.	175.	731.	8772.

1. On the Cost of Smoking Chart, circle the average number of packs you smoke per day, draw a line under the number and straight across the chart.

2. Find the amount you spend per year, depending upon the cost of smoking when and where you read this. If you pay more than $4 a pack, combine two totals to come close to the amount you pay. (For example, In Canada, combine the $4 and $2 totals to get $6 per pack.)

3. Complete the "Cost of Maintaining the Smoking Habit" form (next page).

4. Complete the following calculations:

   $ _____ Annual maintenance cost

   $ _____ Annual cost of tobacco

   ....

   $ _____ Amount you will have saved in one year (without interest. See Interest charts following for compounded amounts.)

5. In your notebook, on the REWARDS page, write your ideas of how you intend to reward yourself with this amount. List new ideas as you think of them—short-term and long-term rewards.

THE COST OF MAINTAINING THE SMOKING HABIT

In addition to the cost of tobacco use, there is a hidden cost of smoking. The cost of the pack or carton is only a part of the money that goes up in smoke! Estimate your own expenditures in the categories listed below. The averages are suggested by a survey of smokers conducted by the Center for the Study of Smoking Behavior.

$ _____ Life insurance premiums—about two times more than non-smokers

$ _____ Loss of earnings due to smoking illnesses. (Five days average/yr; eight days of disability leave/yr)

$ _____ Auto scrapes due to smoking ($50 deductible)

$ _____ Burned clothing due to smoking. Replacement and repair.

$ _____ Burned carpets and furniture

$ _____ Mouthwash, breath mints, flints, lighters, fluid, cough syrup and lozenges, cold medicine

$ _____ Additional dental care (20% more than non-smokers)

$ _____ Additional medical care and prescriptions. (20% more than non-smokers)

$ _____ Extra dry cleaning: clothing, drapes . . .

$ _____ More frequent house, car and office cleaning; more cleaning compounds, air sprays, etc.

©1992, __lyn Rogers, Easton, PA 18042

$ _____ Repainting home/office more frequently

$ _____ Miscellaneous: driving to store for nothing more than cigarettes, etc.

....

$ _____ TOTAL MAINTENANCE COST PER YEAR
(Transfer answer to item #4 in worksheet above)

COST OF SMOKING: COMPOUND INTEREST CHARTS

The following charts demonstrate the magic of compounding interest on the money you will save when you quit smoking—or the money you'd lose if you continue to burn it up in smoke. (Not counting the additional costs of burned clothes, extra dry cleaning, excess insurance for smokers, etc.)

We've used $3 per pack as the model, but cigarettes cost more than that in many countries already. In the United States, it won't be long before $4 to $5 per pack is average. If you live where cigarettes cost more than $3, use these charts as a basis, and add the multiple.

Peter Rogers, who prepared these charts, explains the reasoning behind these assumptions:

0% is straightforward. No interest or inflation, just actual dollars.

4% would approximate long-term inflation, bank savings, and T-bill rates—low or no risk, and perhaps a bit understated on the inflation part.

7% is a good historical average for Treasury bonds; low risk in the long term.

8.5% is a nice blend of common stocks and government bonds—an average of 7% and 10%.

10% approximates the Dow Jones 30 and Standard & Poor's 500 over twenty-plus year stretches.

12.5% is a not unreasonable return in a well-managed growth and income mutual fund over a ten-plus year period.

So, realistically, these are not outrageous rates for long-term investments.

Another way of looking at it—if a person quits smoking in celebration of the birth of a child, they will have saved enough over eighteen years to pay for the child's college!

COST OF SMOKING ESTIMATOR

Cost Per Pack: $3.00
Assumed Investment return if saved: 0.00%
Assumptions: 30 days per month, 12 months per year

Packs/Day			Years Smoked				
	1	3	5	10	20	30	40
1.0	$1,080	$3,240	$5,400	$10,800	$21,600	$32,400	$43,200
1.5	1,620	4,860	8,100	16,200	32,400	48,600	64,800
2.0	2,160	6,480	10,800	21,600	43,200	64,800	86,400
2.5	2,700	8,100	13,500	27,000	54,000	81,000	108,000
3.0	3,240	9,720	16,200	32,400	64,800	97,200	129,600
3.5	3,780	11,340	18,900	37,800	75,600	113,400	151,200
4.0	4,320	12,960	21,600	43,200	86,400	129,600	172,800
4.5	4,860	14,580	24,300	48,600	97,200	145,800	194,400
5.0	5,400	16,200	27,000	54,000	108,000	162,000	216,000

Cost Per Pack: $3.00
Assumed Investment return if saved: 4.00%
Assumptions: 30 days per month, 12 months per year

Packs/Day	Years Smoked						
	1	3	5	10	20	30	40
1.0	$1,100	$3,436	$5,967	$13,252	$33,010	$62,464	$106,377
1.5	1,650	5,155	8,950	19,879	49,515	93,697	159,565
2.0	2,200	6,873	11,934	26,505	66,019	124,929	212,753
2.5	2,750	8,591	14,917	33,131	82,524	156,161	265,941
3.0	3,300	10,309	17,901	39,757	99,029	187,393	319,130
3.5	3,850	12,027	20,884	46,384	115,534	218,626	372,318
4.0	4,400	13,745	23,868	53,010	132,039	249,858	425,506
4.5	4,950	15,464	26,851	59,636	148,544	281,090	478,694
5.0	5,500	17,182	29,835	66,262	165,049	312,322	531,883

Cost Per Pack: $3.00
Assumed Investment return if saved: 7.00%
Assumptions: 30 days per month, 12 months per year

				Years Smoked			
Packs/Day	1	3	5	10	20	30	40
1.0	$1,115	$3,594	$6,443	$15,578	$46,883	$109,797	$236,233
1.5	1,673	5,391	9,665	23,366	70,325	164,696	354,350
2.0	2,231	7,187	12,887	31,155	93,767	219,595	472,466
2.5	2,788	8,984	16,108	38,944	117,208	274,493	590,583
3.0	3,346	10,781	19,330	46,733	140,650	329,392	708,700
3.5	3,904	12,578	22,552	54,522	164,092	384,291	826,816
4.0	4,461	14,375	25,773	62,311	187,534	439,190	944,933
4.5	5,019	16,172	28,995	70,099	210,975	494,088	1,063,049
5.0	5,577	17,969	32,217	77,888	234,417	548,987	1,181,166

Cost Per Pack: $3.00
Assumed Investment return if saved: 8.50%
Assumptions: 30 days per month, 12 months per year

Packs/Day	Years Smoked						
	1	3	5	10	20	30	40
1.0	$1,123	$3,676	$6,700	$16,932	$56,430	$148,564	$363,479
1.5	1,685	5,515	10,050	25,399	84,645	222,845	545,218
2.0	2,246	7,352	13,400	33,865	112,860	297,127	726,957
2.5	2,808	9,190	16,750	42,331	141,075	371,409	908,697
3.0	3,369	11,028	20,099	50,797	169,290	445,691	1,090,436
3.5	3,931	12,865	23,449	59,264	197,505	519,972	1,272,175
4.0	4,492	14,703	26,799	67,730	225,720	594,254	1,453,915
4.5	5,054	16,541	30,149	76,196	253,935	668,536	1,635,654
5.0	5,615	18,379	33,499	84,662	282,150	742,818	1,817,394

Cost Per Pack: $3.00
Assumed Investment return if saved: 10.00%
Assumptions: 30 days per month, 12 months per year

				Years Smoked			
Packs/Day	1	3	5	10	20	30	40
1.0	$1,131	$3,760	$6,969	$18,436	$68,343	$203,444	$569,167
1.5	1,696	5,641	10,454	27,654	102,515	305,166	853,751
2.0	2,262	7,521	13,939	36,872	136,686	406,888	1,138,334
2.5	2,827	9,401	17,423	46,090	170,858	508,610	1,422,918
3.0	3,393	11,281	20,908	55,308	205,030	610,332	1,707,501
3.5	3,958	13,161	24,393	64,526	239,201	712,054	1,992,085
4.0	4,524	15,041	27,877	73,744	273,373	813,776	2,276,669
4.5	5,089	16,922	31,362	82,962	307,544	915,498	2,561,252
5.0	5,655	18,802	34,847	92,180	341,716	1,017,220	2,845,836

Cost Per Pack: $3.00
Assumed Investment return if saved: 12.50%
Assumptions: 30 days per month, 12 months per year

				Years Smoked			
Packs/Day	1	3	5	10	20	30	40
1.0	$1,144	$3,907	$7,450	$21,322	$95,264	$351,685	$1,240,912
1.5	1,716	5,860	11,174	31,983	142,897	527,527	1,861,368
2.0	2,288	7,814	14,899	42,644	190,529	703,370	2,481,824
2.5	2,860	9,767	18,624	53,306	238,161	879,212	3,102,280
3.0	3,432	11,720	22,349	63,967	285,793	1,055,054	3,722,736
3.5	4,004	13,674	26,073	74,628	333,425	1,230,897	4,343,192
4.0	4,576	15,627	29,798	85,289	381,058	1,406,739	4,963,648
4.5	5,148	17,580	33,523	95,950	428,690	1,582,582	5,584,104
5.0	5,720	19,534	37,248	106,611	476,322	1,758,424	6,204,560

Example of Pack Straps #1, 2 and 3

PACK STRAP #1

RECAP	D	D	D	D	D
5	5	5	5	5	5
6	6	6	6	6	6
7	7	7	7	7	7
8	8	8	8	8	8
9	9	9	9	9	9
10	10	10	10	10	10
11	11	11	11	11	11
12	12	12	12	12	12
1	1	1	1	1	1
2	2	2	2	2	2
3	3	3	3	3	3
4	4	4	4	4	4
5	5	5	5	5	5
6	6	6	6	6	6
7	7	7	7	7	7
8	8	8	8	8	8
9	9	9	9	9	9
10	10	10	10	10	10
11	11	11	11	11	11
12	12	12	12	12	12
1	1	1	1	1	1
2	2	2	2	2	2
3	3	3	3	3	3
4	4	4	4	4	4
T	T	T	T	T	T

PACK STRAP #2

2

RECAP	D	D	D	D	D	D	D
5	5	5	5	5	5	5	5
6	6	6	6	6	6	6	6
7	7	7	7	7	7	7	7
8	8	8	8	8	8	8	8
9	9	9	9	9	9	9	9
10	10	10	10	10	10	10	10
11	11	11	11	11	11	11	11
12	12	12	12	12	12	12	12
1	1	1	1	1	1	1	1
2	2	2	2	2	2	2	2
3	3	3	3	3	3	3	3
4	4	4	4	4	4	4	4
6	5	5	5	5	5	5	5
7	6	6	6	6	6	6	6
8	7	7	7	7	7	7	7
9	8	8	8	8	8	8	8
10	9	9	9	9	9	9	9
11	10	10	10	10	10	10	10
12	11	11	11	11	11	11	11
1	12	12	12	12	12	12	12
2	1	1	1	1	1	1	1
3	2	2	2	2	2	2	2
4	3	3	3	3	3	3	3
T	4	4	4	4	4	4	4
	T	T	T	T	T	T	T

PACK STRAP #3

РЕCAP

| D | 5 | 6 | 7 | 8 | 9 | 10 | 11 | 12 | 1 | 2 | 3 | 4 | 5 | 6 | 7 | 8 | 9 | 10 | 11 | 12 | 1 | 2 | 3 | 4 | T |

Countdown to Cutoff

I WILL STOP SMOKING ON

Oct. 27, 1985

TOTAL ②

DAY 7
11 .. Upset /
2 .. Allowed /
4 .. No reason /
7 .. one hr. after dinner /
TOTAL ④

DAY 6
1 .. Before lunch - allowed /
6 .. a desire /
8 .. one hr after dinner /
TOTAL ③

DAY 5
10 .. Bad news ///
1 .. allowed /
3 .. tired /
4 .. Tired + Hungry /
10 .. no reason /
TOTAL ⑦

DAY 4
2 .. no reason /
7 .. no reason /
TOTAL ②

DAY 3
1 .. allowed /
6 .. allowed /
TOTAL ②

DAY 2
10 .. Allowed /
3 .. no reason /
7 .. allowed /
TOTAL ③

DAY 1 (Cut-off Tonight)
6 .. allowed /
1 AM - ///
TOTAL ④

© JR 1986

4
(Example)

Fold

Fold

Countdown to Cut-off

DAY 7	DAY 6	DAY 5
I WILL STOP SMOKING ON _____ 19___		
TOTAL DAY 4	TOTAL DAY 3	TOTAL DAY 2	TOTAL DAY 1 (Cut-off Tonight)
TOTAL	TOTAL	TOTAL	TOTAL

Fold

Fold

© JR 1986

Review this often after you quit—forewarned is forearmed.

PROJECTING FUTURE "HIDDEN" TRIGGERS

SPECIFIC ROUTINES
Emerging from a department
  store or movie theater
A break at a meeting
Waiting rooms
Intermission at a performance
Embarking on a plane trip
"No Smoking" sign goes off
Riding in a taxi cab
Sedentary competition—
  chess, bridge, poker,
  scrabble, backgammon, etc.
Waiting for your turn to bowl
Car breaks down
Stuck in traffic
All night vigil at the hospital

SEASONAL EVENTS
First swim of the season
First ski run of the season
Spring cleaning
Out on the boat, fishing
Golf tournament, tennis, etc.
On line at post office,
  Christmas rush
Filing Income Tax Return
Wedding reception
Attending a football game
Waiting in physician or
  dentist's office for an
  examination
Mowing the lawn, raking
  leaves
Shoveling snow off the
  sidewalk
Home being painted
Final exams/Qualifying exams

SOCIAL TRIGGERS
Attending a big party
Terminating a personal
  relationship
The only one not invited
Being snubbed
The boss and wife are coming
  to dinner
Stranger in town
Embarrassed by a faux pas
Someone you just met offers
  you a cigarette—your
  former brand
Stood up for a date
Cancelling the wedding
Spilled red wine on your
  hostess's heirloom lace
  tablecloth
Friend who smokes moves in
  for a month
First time you have a houseful
  of smoking guests
Showing off, complacent—
  bragging one can't hurt,
  you've got it made

ADRENALINE PUMPING
OVERTIME
Automobile accident
A child in danger
Robbery/Burglary/Mugging
Rescuing a victim
Fire
Escape from danger
Won the lottery
Good news/Bad news/No news

HIDDEN TRIGGERS

EMOTIONAL TRIGGERS
Self pity
Disillusionment
Did poorly on an exam
A fight with a loved one
Financial setback
Learning of a serious illness
Failure
Fighting a deadline
Balancing the checkbook
Request for a raise turned
    down
Boredom
Loss of job (retired/fired)
Job interviews
Loss of a loved one
Loss of a big order
Fear of unknown—an
    operation, new job, move to
    another city
Feeling inadequate
Kept waiting for someone who
    is late
Success (end of striving)
Loss of a pet
Loss of precious property
Loneliness
Ailing parent comes to live
    with you
Kids move away from home

PHYSICAL TRIGGERS
Accident resulting in pain
Resting after biking up a hill
Holiday fragrances (Christmas,
    Thanksgiving, etc.)
Subliminal messages
A strain of music that's tied to
    a former smoking response
No heat in winter, very cold

No air conditioning in
    summer, very hot
Personal encounter with
    someone you used to
    smoke with
Consumed too much alcohol
Hallucinogens (grass, coke,
    etc.)

ADD YOUR OWN

TOOLS TO COPE

Here is a guide to help you deal with those problems you may formerly have dealt with by smoking. The Cigarette didn't help, but it was something you did until you figured out a practical solution—a way to cope.

Now, instead of lighting up in the face of a problem, refer to this guide and review your options. Try to think of other ideas of your own, as well.

First **Decode**—pinpoint the nature of your dissatisfaction. Second—find an immediate solution in the **Distract** column. Third—plan a way to **Repattern** so you don't get caught short the next time.

DECODE	DISTRACT	REPATTERN
Hungry	Oral Gratification Routine. Mouth Spray.	Have a "serious snack" instead of sweets. Also a good weight control.
Angry/ Frustrated	Deep Breathing. Do something physical—bang on a piano or drum.	Resolve to avoid source of anger or frustration in future, or change your approach to it.
Lonely	Call or write a friend or buddy. Reward yourself. Visit someone lonelier than you.	Become involved with people; make yourself important to others. Do someone a favor.
Tired	Take a break and stretch. Deep breathing. Orange Juice/Bouillon.	Get adequate rest at night. Schedule a nap during the day if you can.
Bored/Restless	Do something physical. Refer to REWARDS/ DISTRACTIONS THAT ARE NEITHER COSTLY NOR FATTENING . . . Start some project you've been meaning to get to.	Adult Education classes, new hobby. Add some variety to your daily routine.
Depressed	Do something physical. Fix yourself up—look your best. Have a good cry, and get it over with.	Become involved with people. Check out possibility of water retention. Plan daily rewards.
Worried	Relaxation Ritual. Walk, run—do something physical.	Put problems into perspective. Attack smallest problem first and resolve it.

DECODE	DISTRACT	REPATTERN
Disappointed	Mirror Talk. Reward Yourself.	Plan an alternative strategy ahead of time, just in case. Accept it with a mature attitude—set a new goal.
Feelings Hurt	See REWARDS/ DISTRACTIONS . . . Write in your Log Book about what happened. Read back what you wrote and gain perspective.	Develop a sense of humor. Try to understand the *other* person's needs and motivations.
Indigestion	Antacid—in lozenge or liquid form.	Avoid overeating and highly seasoned foods.
Embarrassed	Remind yourself you're only human. Call on your sense of humor.	Don't be so concerned with what others might think of you . . . they are more concerned with themselves. Rely on your new sense of self-esteem.
Familiar Trigger	Recognize it as a former smoking situation. Observe how nonsmokers handle themselves.	Anticipate trigger situations ahead of time—strip them of their power—diffuse their impact.
Self-Pity	Mirror Talk. Try laughter—chances are you're taking yourself too seriously.	Learn to say "no". Plan daily rewards.
About to Light Up	Deep breathing. Smell your Butt Jar. Smell a smoker. Call a buddy.	Review those ego reasons for quitting. Eliminate self-pity. Nurture your positive attitude.
Tension	Relaxation Ritual. Take a hot shower or bath. Go for a walk or a swim.	Increase Vitamin B_1 in form of whole grains, wheat germ. Try to avoid tension-producing confrontations as much as possible.
Difficulty Concentrating	Deep breathing. Take a walk. Come back to it after you've taken a break.	Attack the task during more productive time of day for you. Examine why—if boring material, try to get to something more absorbing.
Stress/Pressure	Deep breathing. Exercise—diffuse stress by activating whole body. Walk away from the situation.	Learn to control your response to stress producing situations—be flexible, do what's comfortable for you.

DECODE	DISTRACT	REPATTERN
Insomnia	Relaxation Ritual. Warm milk with honey. Read something supremely boring.	Change hour of retiring. Don't permit any daytime napping. No caffeine after dinner.
Gained Weight	Be mature—consider it a temporary inconvenience for a permanent improvement. Do something physical.	Go on a diet. Repattern your eating as you repatterned your smoking behavior.
Rushed	Take your time, in spite of circumstances. Deep breathing. Don't be afraid to tell someone you need more time.	Try to start earlier. Anticipate situations that might slow you down, and try to circumvent them or allow time for them.
Feeling Bloated (Fluid Retention)	Elevate your legs. Drink water (if reduced salt intake). Approach it positively as a temporary Symptom of Recovery.	Make yourself knowledgeable about high sodium foods and avoid salt.
Nibbling Too Much	Chew on ginger root or clove. Drink Water. Oral Gratification Routine.	Pinpoint your bad eating habits and resolve to change them. Restock your kitchen with sensible snacks.
Completion of a Pleasurable event	Count your blessings! Smile at your good fortune. Remind yourself that "one *will* hurt."	Fully enjoy the "event"—nothing more is needed.

Instant Go

PICK UP IDEAS . . . FOR ENERGY . . . APPEARANCE . . . ATTITUDE!

Now that you're an ex-smoker, try the following for—

1. INSTANT START IN THE MORNING:
   - Stretch . . . slowly . . . gently.
   - Stand TALL!
   - Shower Power (needle sharp—lukewarm).

2. INSTANT TENSION RELIEF & GOOD CIRCULATION:
   - Three deep down breaths.
   - Bend from the waist—hang there like a rag doll.
   - Walk everywhere!
   - Don't slouch!

3. INSTANT ENERGY AND PICKUP:
   - Stretch . . . slowly . . . deliberately.
   - Smile!
   - Increase Vitamin B complex.
   - Eat lightly every three hours instead of heavy 3 times a day.
   - Splash cold water on face, neck and wrists.
   - Try hot bouillon or ice cold orange juice.

4. INSTANT SOUL SATISFIER:
   - Smile a warm, sincere smile at the next ten people with whom you have dealings.
   - Sincerely appreciate all the efforts of all the people who are working for you and with you . . . AND TELL THEM SO!
   - Say something genuinely nice to someone at least once each day.

5. INSTANT SLEEPING PILL:
   - Do Relaxation Ritual.
   - Hop into bed—flat on back, knee bent (changes curvature of spine so no backache).
   - Breath deeply into diaphragm 5 times while reciting a positive, pleasant statement endlessly . . . "TOMORROW WILL BE A GOOD DAY" . . . or "I'M SO GLAD I DON'T SMOKE ANYMORE", etc.
   - Try focusing on one event likely to occur the next day which pleases you, or which you anticipate with great enthusiasm.
   - Dwelling on the mistakes of today or the fears of tomorrow doesn't create relaxation . . . and can't solve anything either!!!!

FINAL QUESTIONNAIRE:
YOU CAN STOP SMOKING

Let me know how you're doing. Send this questionnaire, or drop me a note or letter to the following address.

Jacquelyn Rogers
Box 550
Easton, Pa 18044-0550

Tell me about yourself somewhat as follows:

Dear Jackie,

I smoked _____ packs of cigarettes/pipes/cigars a day for _____ years. I am _____ years old and started to smoke when I was _____ years old, because _____
_____

Regarding nicotine replacement:
☐ I have used the _____ brand nicotine patch since
_____ (date)
☐ I no longer use it because _____
_____
_____

☐ I'm still on it because _____
_____
_____

☐ I read your book and stopped smoking on _____

☐ I haven't quit yet but intend to—or don't intend to—or etc.)

☐ I'm ready to quit but I'd like to do SmokEnders seminar or use the audiocassette program, so I'll call them: 800-828-4357.

My reasons for quitting are _____
_____
_____
_____
_____
_____
_____

The book helped me (in what way?) or it didn't help me, because

_____

_____

_____

_____

_____

☐ I bought the book because _____

_____

_____

(or it was given to me by someone who loves me—or I pinched it
from a friend—or someone I loves smokes and I wanted to know
how to help him/her—or I'm a health professional and want more
information—or I'm a SmokEnder graduate and wanted to read
it—or I quit smoking previously and wanted reinforcement, or
etc.)

I bought the book at _____

☐ Send me information about the Facilitator's Guide.

My comments/suggestions are: _____

_____

_____

_____

_____

_____

_____

_____

Name _____

Address _____

City _____ State ____ Zip ____

Phone ____/_____ (day) ____/_____ (eve)